Contents

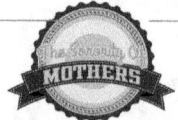

Introduction

Written by: A Sorority of Mothers

This book contains proven steps and strategies on how to **understand what being a future mom (and a new mom) is all about.** Many times, people don't tell you about the worst things you should be expecting to live through when pregnant. Not informing yourself on what to expect is one of the worst things you can do. Truth be told, pregnancy is far from being a fantasy-like dream come true and there are certain things you should really be prepared for. Some of them may be well known to you. But others are so well concealed by most of the "specialty" books that it all seems like a piece of cake. It isn't!

Pregnancy is not easy to take on. It will require you to change things about your everyday life and it will change you forever. Yet every single minute of effort and change you put into this is going to be so worth it! Being a parent is not an easy thing, but it is definitely one of the most rewarding experiences one can get from life. Being able to hold your baby, to help him grow healthy and beautiful, to guide his steps in life, to see that he eventually turns out very well – all these things can't be put in words and all those who are already parents know it. The responsibility of parenting is great and it all starts with your pregnancy.

If you have just found out that you are pregnant, this is one of the best books to read, not because we will present you with beautiful lies, but because we will present you with the **truth** as it is from a mother's perspective. We will give you facts, helpful tips, current information on what to expect; sometimes unbearably beautiful, sometimes unpleasant, but always part of a future parent's life. **Thanks again for downloading this book,** we hope you enjoy it!

A Sorority of Mothers is a gathering place for mothers' online www.asororityofmothers.com this sorority gathers to share their experiences and tips. The purpose is to help future mothers and experienced mothers alike. The goal of the Sorority is to aide each member in motherhood, and to become the Best mother (Mommy) possible. **Motherhood is not easy and does not come with instructions**. What makes our books great is that you are not getting one person's perspective but the facts and viewpoints from several women who have all had different experiences during pregnancy and motherhood. We have written this book to aide mothers with questions that they may have, share tips, and prepare them for the upcoming months. We all sincerely thank you for your purchase of this book.

Please enjoy this book. If you have any questions, please email us @

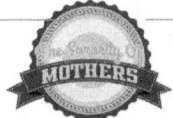

We have members there to answer questions at all times. Thank you!

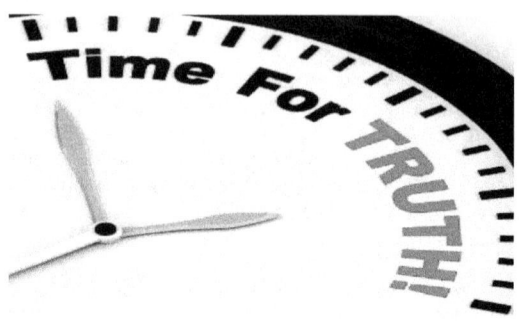

Pregnancy Facts

- Half a million babies are born in the USA to a teen mother
- About 15% of all mothers will be diagnosed with post **partum depression**
- 90% of all babies will be born within 2 weeks of their due date.
- Morning sickness will occur in about 73% of all pregnancies.
- About 4% of pregnancies will result in twins.
- 2013: Top girl baby name- 1.Sophia 2.Emma 3.Olivia
- 2013: Top boy baby name- 1.Jackson 2.Aiden 3.Liam

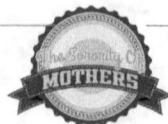

- About 4 million babies are born in the USA each year.
- Average age of a first time mother in the USA is 25.1 years old.
- The most popular day for pregnant women to give birth surprisingly is Tuesday.
- The least popular day to give birth is Sunday.
- 30% of women gain 21-30 pounds during pregnancy
- 25% of women gain 31-40 pounds during pregnancy
- 21% of women gain more than 40 pounds during pregnancy
- 16% of women gain 11-20 pounds during pregnancy
- About 1 in 10 women smoke during their pregnancy
- Caesarean delivers occur in about 35% of all deliveries
- 1050 male babies are born to every 1000 female babies
- Premature birth occurs in about 12% of all deliveries
- The average US birth weight is about 7lbs
- The average UK birth weight is 7.1lbs
- About 10% of all pregnancies will end in miscarriage
- The longest pregnancy was 375days! Woman gave birth to a normal and healthy baby girl, which she named Penny.
- Studies have shown that your sense of smell will increase about 30%!
- Your feet can grow around one shoe size larger.
- About 4% of the female population in the USA is pregnant right now.
- About 30% of teens in the USA become pregnant.
- Every 87 seconds a women will die from childbirth
- While pregnant, you will need to add about 300 calories a day to your diet.
- A baby is born every 3 seconds worldwide
- During the first year, average parents in the USA will spend about

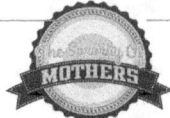

$7,000 dollars on services.

- Morning sickness can be reduced with small portion meals.
- Your blood volume will increase by up to 50% during pregnancy.
- The oldest mother ever registered was 69 years old!
- Only about 6% of mothers actually give birth on their official due date.
- In most cases, women don't show until the end of their 11th week.
- In the second half of your pregnancy, you will pee over a full liter a day!
- Women having Cesarean sections have tripled over the past 10 years!
- Females are born with all of their eggs for their lifetime, while boys don't produce sperm until around 12.
- 91% of women will experience some sort of skin change during pregnancy.
- Each year the average weight of a baby has increased for the past two decades.
- *Normal Labor can begin 2 weeks before the due date*
- *Also labor can begin up to 2 weeks after the due date*
- *In your first stage of Labor, your cervix dilates and thins*
- *In your second stage of labor, it is time to push!*
- *The second stage begins when you are dilated to 10cm.*
- *The third stage is when the placenta and membranes are delivered.*
- *You may not be allowed to eat during labor, be prepared.*
- *A lot of people will look between your legs at your private area!*
- *While pushing, you may have an accident? (If you know what we mean?)*
- *Women in the B.C. era gave birth on stools.*
- *Before effective painkillers, women would drink alcohol during labor!*
- *Your uterus will expand up to 500 times the normal size!*
- *Studies show that tall women are more likely to have twins.*
- *Your baby will not feel the umbilical cord being cut.*

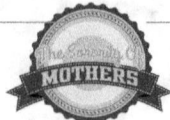

- *The average number of days being pregnant is 280.*
- *The ratio of stillborn births is 1.5 females to 1.0 male.*
- *The last organ that your baby will develop is their lungs.*
- *Your baby won't develop fingerprints until it reaches 3 months old.*
- *Every human being in the world has been a single cell organism for at least an hour!*
- *At one month old should feed every three to four hours*
- *Breastfeed babies will wake more often*
- *Breastfeed babies do not get as much volume in feeding.*
- *Babies do cluster feed.*
- *They may want to eat every hour during the day.*
- *The will experience 3-5 wet diapers a day.*
- *A baby may not poop for up to 5 days.*
- *Between 1-3 months the baby will begin to recognize your face.*
- *1-3 month babies will still have the startle reflex. (Loud Noise)*
- *Tummy time is good for their strength.*
- *Babies don't need water until 4 months.*

The Fantasy: What New Moms Think Pregnancy Is Like

When finding out about the new pregnancy, most of the new mothers already picture themselves crying tears of joy at the sight of their son's or daughter's college diploma.

Not yet, though. You've got more than two decades until then, out of which the first couple of years will be completely life changing.

Pregnancy is wonderful on its own: the mere fact that you are able to *create life* is a miracle if you think of it this way. But making sure that the life you give birth to gets on the right path is a completely different matter.

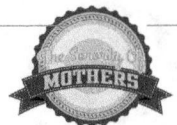

A lot of new moms think that, outside of their first months' morning sickness and dizziness, everything will go just fine. And really, they are not to be blamed for this: with so many movies out there picturing ever-laughing pretty dressed pregnant ladies, there seems to be no reason why you should think your own pregnancy shouldn't go the same way.

The truth is a bit more complex than movies show it, actually. After all, who in the world would ever watch a movie about ladies complaining about extra weight, about the heaviness of carrying a baby bump, about the fact that maternity clothes are downright expensive and about the fact that baby fat will not go away as soon as you get out of the hospital? Nobody.

And, to top that, celebrities aren't helping much either. You see them everywhere: new mothers who have just given birth and look as if they were 18: slim, toned up, gorgeous and perfect.

In addition to the outside changes pregnant bodies go through, there is a series of hormonal and psychological changes not many new moms expect. Of course, you may expect to have odd feelings every once in a while and some of you may even expect to feel anxious and downright scared. But you will most likely not expect to seriously question your decision of being a mother, you will most likely not expect to suddenly feel the burden of an entire human life hanging on your shoulders and you may not expect the huge range of feelings that may overwhelm you.

Yes, pregnant ladies do get priority in the bus, at the supermarket and they do get more attention. Everybody will feel like pampering and protecting you. You will enjoy buying baby clothes, feeling your kid kick his little feet in your belly and decorating the baby's room.

But there is so much more to pregnancy than this and you should definitely be prepared for it all. Hopefully, the following chapters will cover most of the things you should know.

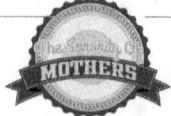

Pregnancy Myths Busted

Once you tell everyone that you are pregnant, you will most likely be flooded by a long series of pieces of advice and myths that are not always as true as some think.
In fact, there are so many myths and superstitions related to pregnancy that it can get downright confusing, especially for the new parents out there. It is very important that you know exactly what to believe and what not to believe because it can affect the way your entire pregnancy will go from now on. This is why we have put together a series of myths related to this very special moment in one's life. Read on and find out about the most commonly encountered misconceptions about pregnancy that are as false as it can get.

Flying

Some people believe that pregnant women are not allowed to fly during their first and during their last semester of pregnancy, but that is not completely true. There is no health-related reason that should prevent you from getting on a flight (none at all, actually). However, some of the companies don't allow pregnant women to fly during the last semester because they fear the women may get into labor (and this can lead to forced landings and ruining upholstery as well).

Smoked Salmon

Some women believe that they are not allowed to eat smoked salmon when they are pregnant, but this is, again, not true. As a matter of fact, it is completely the opposite: you *should* eat salmon because it is rich in Omega-3 fatty acids which are crucial both for the health of your own body and for the health of your baby as well. Even more than that, it has been proven that salmon can help babies come to birth healthier and...smarter as well.

Ridiculous Myths

There are some pregnancy-related myths out there that are downright ludicrous. For instance, some say that pregnant women should not touched polished furniture. Other people say that pregnant women should not have sex, lift their hands above their head, that they shouldn't dry their hair, that they shouldn't sleep on the right side, which they shouldn't eat hot dogs and the list goes on and on... All these myths are, as you may have suspected, false. There is absolutely no reason in the world why you should not eat hot dogs (as long as they are well-made), why you shouldn't blow-dry your hair or why you shouldn't sit on your

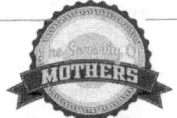

own couch.

Walking and Labor

Another myth that is quite commonly encountered out there is related to walking and to the fact that it can make labor come faster. No matter how disappointing this news must be to you, the truth is that there is nothing out there that can make labor come or go faster. Your body is the only one who knows just when it will come and how long it will last.

Eating, Nutrition and Weight

Some of the women out there say that they should be eating for two. If you follow that rule, it is very likely that you will gain a lot of weight. In truth, a pregnant woman needs only about 300 calories more than she eats on average. After all, it is a *baby* that will not weigh much more than 7-8 pounds that you are "carrying" in you, not a full-grown adult who should get the same nutritional intake as you do. As for the weight of the baby, bigger is not always better. In fact, it has been shown that babies that are born with a higher than average weight are at more risk to develop diabetes.

Exercising

It is believed that exercising is bad for the fetus. As a matter of fact, as long as you do special pregnancy exercises, your fetus will most likely be born healthier and with a bigger brain. So, it is perfectly fine to attend a pregnant ladies' gym class.

The Shape of the Belly

Some say that the shape of a pregnant woman's belly can predict on whether she will have a girl or a boy (pointy bellies are for boys and flatter bellies are for girls). Yet, this has absolutely no actual grounds to be based on. The shape of your baby bump has absolutely nothing to do with the sex of your child! In many cultures, there are other ways of "predicting" the sex of the baby. For instance, in Easter Europe women throw a needle on the floor and if the pregnant woman bends down to pick it up in a certain way, she will give birth to a boy. Again, as you would probably suspect it, this is complete non-sense.

What and How You Eat Will Not Affect the Fetus

If you believe that your dietary habits during the pregnancy will not affect the fetus, you are very wrong. Actually, your eating habits can certainly affect the baby. For

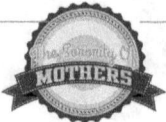

instance, eating too much junk food and unhealthy food could be the first step towards childhood obesity for your baby. Make sure you eat healthy and that you maintain your health because it can really affect your baby's health too.

Seatbelts

This is probably one of the most dangerous pregnancy-related myths out there. Many people think that pregnant women should not be wearing a seatbelt, but this is completely and utterly wrong. You should **definitely** wear your seatbelt every single time you ride in a car! Of course, you should make sure that it doesn't cross your belly, but that can be easily done by placing the upper belt on your chest and by placing the lower one right below the belly.

Hair Coloring

This is not an actual myth, but up to the moment it has not been confirmed or infirmed either. There is not much of a reason why you shouldn't be able to dye your hair. However, considering the fact that hair dyes contain powerful chemicals you could breathe in, it is best to actually avoid this one. Your hair will look perfectly fine if it's not dyed for the following 9 months as well!

Cleaning the Floors and Labor

All right, this is another very funny and completely illogical one: they say that you can induce labor if you start sweeping your floors and cleaning your house. While there may be ways in which one can induce labor, they are related to actual science and medicine and not to any kind of huge house cleanup you may want to do. If you feel that you need to clean the house a bit, then do it, but do make sure you don't strain yourself too much because that will not induce you labor, but it can put you and your baby to danger.

Alcohol

Drinking alcohol has been a No-No since bible times. "Behold, thou shalt conceive and bear a son; and now drink no wine nor strong drink, neither any unclean thing." (Judges 13:7).

Alcohol can lead to some very scary risks. Number one is Fetal Alcohol Syndrome (FAS). Babies with FAS can be slow to arouse and behave sluggish in general. Babies born to heavy drinkers have more than twice to chance of developing physical abnormalities. Some examples are a thin upper lip, and a short nose. The last trimester is the most critical in development. Heavy drinking during this

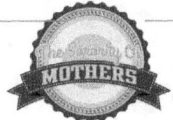

trimester can lead to heart defects, small heads, distortion of joints, and may show mental retardation, and slowed motor development.

Recent studies have shown that even moderate drinking can be very damaging. The best route to take is to not drink at all.

Cigarettes

Smoking cigarettes will harm the fetus. The two key elements are nicotine and carbon monoxide. These two elements can interfere with the supply of oxygen to the fetus. With the reduction of oxygen, the baby's heart must beat faster than normal. One cigarette can cause the baby's heart to beat 20% faster than normal. It will continue at this high rate for about 15-20 minutes after the cigarette has been finished.

Smoking during pregnancy has been linked to reduced birth weight, increased risk of miscarriage, prematurity, and a higher rate of infant mortality at birth. Smoking has also been linked to many other risks. Structural abnormalities, increased concentration of carbon monoxide in both maternal and fetal bloodstreams, and central nervous system damages to name a few.

From all of the Sorority to you, **please**, at all cost, do not smoke while you are pregnant!

Pregnancy Diet Concerns

Paying attention to your diet before you plan to conceive can reduce your risk of having a baby born with a birth defect that affects the brain or spinal cord (neural tube defects), such as spina bifida or anencephaly. The first eight weeks after conception are the most crucial time in your baby's development. By the eighth week, the developing fetus has a complete nervous system, a beating heart, a fully formed digestive system, and the beginnings of facial features. Neural tube defects occur during the first month of pregnancy when the neural tube is forming. As many as half of all pregnancies are unplanned, so many women, including female athletes, don't realize that they are pregnant at this time. Weight gain can be minimal during these first few weeks, and a woman may attribute a late or missed menstrual period to hard training efforts or the stress associated with competitions.

Consuming 400 micrograms a day of the B vitamin foliate or folic acid will help your developing baby form and develop new and normal body tissues. (Foliate is

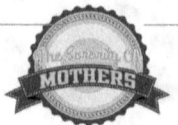

used when the vitamin is found naturally in foods; folic acid is used when it is found in supplements.) Natural sources of foliate include legumes, such as lentils and dried beans, leafy green vegetables (especially spinach and broccoli), whole grains, orange juice, and some fortified breakfast cereals. Grain products, such as breads, pasta, rice, cornmeal, and enriched flours, are now being fortified with small amounts of folic acid too. Nevertheless, most women do not consume adequate amounts of foliate in their diet.

If you're contemplating pregnancy, see your doctor before you try to conceive and begin taking a prenatal vitamin–mineral supplement as directed to obtain the folic acid that you need. Because many pregnancies are unplanned, the March of Dimes, a research organization that studies birth defects, recommends that all women of childbearing age, whether planning to become pregnant or not, take a multivitamin with 400 micrograms of folic acid daily and eat foliate-rich foods. (Excessive levels of vitamin A can be toxic to a developing baby. Avoid taking a daily multivitamin containing more than 5,000 IU of vitamin A.)
Abstaining from alcohol makes sense too. No safe level of alcohol consumption has been determined for pregnant women. Consuming limited amounts of alcohol after conception but before becoming aware that you're pregnant shouldn't cause distress. Regularly consuming alcoholic beverages, however, does affect the developing fetus. Having one to two drinks per day can result in a smaller baby. Drinking greater amounts can lead to birth defects associated with fetal alcohol syndrome. The earlier you eliminate alcohol, the better off your baby will be.

The First Trimester and What You Should Expect Now

The first trimester can sometimes be the most difficult one to handle for many women out there. Most of the things that happen to your body now are also signs of pregnancy and you may be familiar with some of them at least. This chapter is dedicated to explaining some of the most commonly encountered pregnancy symptoms women experience during the very first trimester. Hopefully, what is written here will help you get through everything a bit more easily.

Nausea, Vomiting and Morning Sickness

This is probably one of the first pregnancy signs and it is one of the most commonly encountered symptoms as well. Many women feel the so-called "morning sickness" throughout the first 3 months of pregnancy, but some may have such symptoms later on as well. What is interesting about this symptom is related to the fact that "morning sickness" does not always happen in the morning and that many women experience it in the afternoon, at night or at any other

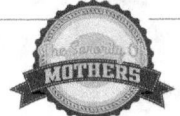

moment of the day. Even more than that, there is no actual research on whether or not more women feel the sickness in the morning or not.

In most of the cases, some sort of food or odor, which may prevent you from eating, triggers the morning sickness. However, you should make sure that you don't force yourself into eating something because that could get you even sicker. Do eat crackers and this kind of "neutral" foods and make sure that you keep yourself hydrated with clear liquids (water, clear soda and so on).

Listening to your body can be an amazing thing. If you notice that you feel nauseous or sick at a specific time of the day, remember to rest and keep yourself away from food then. Also, if you notice that a particular kind of food triggers these reactions in your body, keep yourself away from them as well.

It is very important that you don't take any kind of medication (not even of the over-the-counter type) without prior medical consultation. There are pharmaceutical remedies for nausea and vomiting, and they may not be harmful, but you really have to be 100% certain about it, so following the doctor's advice is the very best way to go around this.

In addition to medication, there are a lot of home remedies you can try to alleviate morning sickness. For instance, peppermint tea may help and so can lemon water. Also, ginger-based products are quite commonly known to fight nausea as well. Some women claim that heated blankets, taking a walk, 2 lavender oil dropped on the pillow and other such things helped them too. If you notice that something appears to make you feel better, remember it and try it when you feel sick again.

Early Pregnancy Signs

- **You may have tender breast and nipples.** You may notice an achy feeling in your breast.
- **Darkened Areolas** are another sign of early pregnancy. They may even increase in diameter.
- **Spotting** is the most common sign seen in women.
- You may begin to notice some **tiny bumps around the Areolas**.
- **Extreme Fatigue** and exhaustion is very common.
- **Frequent Urination** will usually occur about 2-3 weeks after conception.
- **Sensitivity with your smell** is a very common sign in pregnancy.
- **Extreme Bloating** will occur very early after fertilization.
- **Frequent Nausea**, and this is one of the worst signs.
- **Missed Period** is obvious, but it is a real sign!

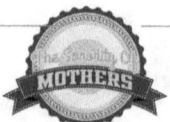

Top 10 Foods to Avoid during Pregnancy

Pregnancy and carrying new life is a wonderful experience for any woman to have! The joy of carrying a precious baby inside of you is hard to put into words! Those nine months of pregnancy are very important for a mother. It is a time when a woman must focus on taking excellent care of herself and her baby. One of the essential keys to taking care of yourself during pregnancy involves the foods you eat. There are a lot of healthy food options that will provide vitamins and minerals that are beneficial to mother and baby. But, there are a certain foods that need to be avoided during a woman's pregnancy. Please continue reading to find out the top ten foods that should be avoided during pregnancy.

1. Raw Sea Food

Raw seafood is best if avoided as it contains harmful parasites that affect the growing fetus. Raw fish may possibly contain three food born pathogens: toxoplasma, listeria monocytogenes, and salmonella enterica. Not to mention that uncooked fish may contain elements of worms or eggs. These are definitely things you want to avoid putting in your body. There is some limited sushi that can still be eaten while pregnant. The best rule of thumb is to only eat fully cooked fish and meat in general. It is not worth the possible risk to baby.

2. Fish High in Mercury

Fish is a high source of protein and omega – 3 fatty acids essential during pregnancy; but certain fish that have high levels of mercury can be very harmful to a growing baby. Mercury is a byproduct of coal-burning plants that disrupts the development of a growing child's brain and nervous system. It is also important to avoid fish that have been caught for sport in a lake or pond because the may contain industrial pollutants that can be harmful to baby. So eat fish, like salmon or shrimp, in limited amounts and be sure to avoid specific fish that are known to have high levels of mercury inside of them.

3. Undercooked Poultry, Meat & Eggs

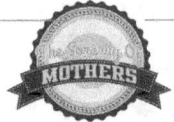

Undercooked or raw poultry, meat or eggs may be contaminated with coliform bacteria, toxoplasmosis, and salmonella. These bacteria can be very harmful to baby and affect their development and growth. To be safe the best way to avoid these harmful bacteria is to ensure that all poultry, meat, and eggs are cooked properly to keep baby safe.

4. Unwashed Vegetables & Fruits

It is important thoroughly wash any fruits and vegetables being eaten. Unwashed fruits and vegetables may contain the bacteria toxoplasmosis. This bacterium is not just a danger to baby, but also to you so make sure to wash all fruit and vegetables.

5. Over Consumption of Vitamin A

Vitamin A is an important vitamin to take during pregnancy. It is important because it directly plays a role in baby's embryonic growth; which involves development of heart, lungs, kidneys, eyes, bones, circulatory, respiratory, and central nervous system. With that being said it is also important to not over consume on Vitamin A. High levels can cause birth defects and liver toxicity. The recommended amount of Vitamin A for women 19 and older should not exceed more than 770 micrograms RAE of Vitamin A per day. The best precaution is to get with your doctor to ensure that daily limit of Vitamin A is reached for baby's healthy development.

6. Caffeine

Caffeine is a substance found in a variety of drinks, foods and these days numerous diet pills and diet aids. It is commonly found inside of soft drinks and coffee, but these are just two of the many sources of caffeine that you will find. People use caffeine for a variety of reasons, even to lose weight, but as we just mentioned it is most commonly used as a source of energy and alertness. It is a stimulant, causing an increase in the central nervous system, thus producing alertness and energy effects within a very short time frame. Caffeine is a crystalline xanthine alkaloid, which can be derived from leaves, seeds and in some fruits of a plant. Inside of these things the caffeine acts as a pesticide that will kill several different insects. Humans consume caffeine that is derived from the coffee bean, kola nut and several others. While considered a drug, it is legal for use, and amazingly, about 90% of all Americans report they use some form of the stimulant every single day. Caffeine withdrawals are possible to experience by

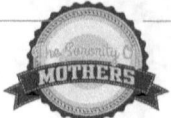

individuals who are heavy users of caffeine if it is abruptly taken away. Those withdrawal symptoms are also different with each person who is experiencing them, and can range from jitters and nervousness to being unable to sleep or eat without the stimulant. Again, the withdrawals are likely to occur only when there is a heavy usage of the substance.

It is very important to **limit** caffeine intake during pregnancy. Too much caffeine can cause miscarriages, especially in the first trimester. When you consume a high amount of caffeine it results in water and calcium lose. Besides just miscarriages, caffeine has also been associated with premature birth, low birth weight and withdrawal symptoms. So remember not to consume more caffeine than needed.

7. Herbal Tea

Drinking herbal tea should be avoided, except for teas that are approved by your doctor. Herbal tea does have caffeine, which increases risk of birth defects.

8. Alcohol

Not for any reason should alcohol be consumed at all during pregnancy. It can cause serious and fatal damage to baby. The side effects of too much alcohol being consumed are permanent damage, brain damage, Fetal Alcohol Syndrome, and other developmental damage. Alcohol also increases the chances of a miscarriage or stillbirth. It is important to know that this includes avoidance after pregnancy especially if you are breast-feeding.

9. Unpasteurized Juice

Unpasteurized juice doesn't protect against harmful bacterial, including salmonella and E. coli. It is important to look at labels and read the warnings to ensure that your juice is pasteurized and your baby is protected. Keep in mind it is perfected safe to make homemade juice for consumption.

10. Unpasteurized Dairy Products

Dairy products such as milk, cheese, and dairy contain bacteria called listeria monocytogenes, which cause foodborne illness such as listeriosis. It is very

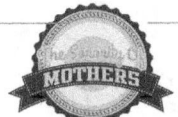

important to ensure that any dairy products consumed have been pasteurized. Always read the label to confirm before purchasing. Listeria affects the growing fetus and causes developmental problems. It can be as serious as causing a miscarriage, still born, or other serious health problems. For the protection of baby, ensure that this food is not consumed during pregnancy.

Shortness of Breath

Another quite common symptom in pregnancy is shortness of breath. Probably due to the fact that your lungs and your entire body are trying to accommodate themselves to the changes the pregnancy brings in, you may feel that you are running out of breath. The best thing to do is to simply sit and breathe in. If you know you suffer from asthma, or if you notice other symptoms this disease may come with, visit your doctor as soon as possible.

Indigestion and Heartburn

Many women experience indigestion and heartburn during their first trimester as well. If you have these symptoms as well, try to avoid eating acid-rich foods, juices and sauces because these are connected to these symptoms. It is also important that you avoid eating anything before you go to sleep. If your symptoms persist even after doing these things, visit the doctor.

Back Pain

It is quite normal to experience back pain during the first trimester as well. Your body's center of gravity will move forward, which means that you will start bending down and which can lead to back pain. Even more, the body will start secreting hormones that are mean to loosen the ligaments and to stretch out the pelvic bone so that you can accommodate the baby and this can sometimes lead to back pain as well. Placing a pillow to support the lower back when working at a desk, taking breaks to stretch, doing some stretching exercises and paying attention to your posture can really go a long way when it comes to this symptom.

Fatigue

It is perfectly normal that you feel overly tired when you are pregnant. After all, your body is making huge efforts to adjust to the new situation. While you cannot prevent fatigue moments, you can however expect them and adjust your schedule accordingly. Your life will indeed change over the course of the following 9 months, but it will all be absolutely worth it!

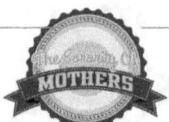

Stress

It is also normal that you feel stressed during your pregnancy (and not just in the first trimester). You *are* going to bear a huge responsibility on your shoulders. However, try to keep the bad kind of stress (the counterproductive one) at bay because the baby can suffer as a consequence of it.

Complexion Changes

Many new pregnant women look as if they shined, and this is due to hormones that are released by the body. However, some women experience a darkening of the skin and this is also related to hormones (too much progesterone and estrogen). The face, the area around the belly button and other parts of the body may experience hyper pigmentation. While there is no actual way to prevent this from happening, you should rest assured that your skin will come back to normal once you have the baby.

Breast Enlargement and Discomfort

Once your body "finds out" that you are pregnant, you will experience breast enlargement as well. This happens because they will want to be able to lactate once the baby is delivered. Again, there is not much you can do about this other than wearing supportive bras. Also, if the skin cracks or becomes irritated, you should get some ointments and treat it with them.

Anemia

A lot of women develop something similar to a "physiologic" anemia during their first trimester. This doesn't happen because the woman is lacking any kind of nutrients, but because her body will start producing much more plasma and less red cells, which leads to a deficiency in the body. It is important that you treat this kind of anemia if it occurs in your case and your doctor can help you by prescribing prenatal vitamin supplements.

Bleeding

This may seem scary to many of you, but the truth is that ¼ of the pregnant women experience it in the first trimester of their pregnancy. If you see spots of blood, then you should not panic because it is a sign that the embryo has been implanted in the uterus. However, any kind of bleeding that may appear to be rather excessive (and especially when it is associated with stomach cramps and abdominal pain) should make you consult your physician as soon as possible. A lot of blood could be the sign of a miscarriage or even of a pregnancy that has

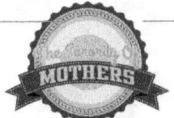

been implanted outside of the uterus.

Vaginal Discharge

It is normal to see a white discharge, but make sure that you don't use a tampon for it because that could get germs in your vagina. However, if the discharge is green, yellow, transparent and excessive or if it smells odd, you should consult with your doctor as soon as possible.

Food Cravings

Again, this is a very commonly known symptom out there and it is perfectly normal to feel it as well. As long as your cravings are not something outrageous or very unhealthy, you can indulge on them. However, the common belief according to which the baby will not develop properly if you don't satisfy your cravings is just a myth.

Urination

You may also notice that you will have to go to the bathroom more frequently than you normally go. This happens because the uterus is slowly increasing its size and it will start putting pressure on your bladder as well. Whatever you do though, don't decrease the amount of liquids you're getting because you really need to keep yourself properly hydrated no matter what.

Mood Swings

It is normal that you experience sudden mood swings as well. Your body is going through a lot of changes and your hormones will be unbalanced, so feeling sad or depressed out of the blue can happen. If it does, make sure that you talk to someone about your feelings because it can really help.

Weight Gain

Now, one of the main things new moms think of when they find out they are pregnant is that they are going to gain a lot of weight and that they will need to get rid of it. Sure, being overweight is not just a matter of fitting into a pair of skinny jeans, but also a matter of actual health so you will want to make sure that you do

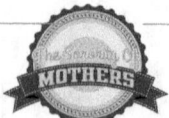

drop it. Normally, you shouldn't put on more than 3-6 pounds in the first trimester so do consult with a doctor if you notice that you have gained a lot more than that. Even if you do keep the weight gain within normal limits, don't expect to return to your shape as soon as you deliver. Same as with any other kind of weight loss program, it will take some time to shed the extra pounds in a healthy way.

Also, remember that while too much extra weight is not a healthy sign, too little extra weight can be a bad sign as well. If you notice that you haven't put on weight or if you notice that you have lost weight, do consult with your medical professional as soon as possible!

There may be many other symptoms that appear in the first trimester of pregnancy, but these are the most commonly encountered ones and knowing about them can be really helpful. It is important that you keep yourself as calm and as sensible as possible when it comes to all these symptoms and that you follow your instinct if you feel that something is wrong. It is better to talk with a doctor and convince yourself that you are in perfect health than not to do it and suffer the consequences.

Understanding Miscarriage

Miscarriage happens to 30% to 40% of all conceptions. Miscarriage is a chance chromosomal or genetic abnormality in the embryo. That means that the embryo has more chromosomes than what should be there. Most miscarriages happen before the woman even knows that she is pregnant. 15% to 20% of miscarriages happen when the woman knows that she is pregnant.

Other factors that play a role in miscarriage are drug use, smoking, excess drinking, Listeria (found in uncooked meats and eggs), also hormonal or structural abnormalities in the mothers (over the age of 35), lupus, and thyroid disease. It does not always happen, but they are factors that come into play.

It is stated that 85% of pregnancies after a miscarriage end with a healthy full term baby, when you decide you want to try again.

15% to 20% of pregnancies end in miscarriage. The causes are not exactly what they say. But they believe that miscarriages happen because of drug use, smoking, excess drinking, etc. Having a miscarriage can cause psychological damage. So women who do lose their baby have to take counseling just to be able to function.

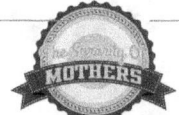

Second Trimester and What You Should Expect Now

Baby bumps are not very obvious during the first trimester, but it is a high chance that people will start noticing yours during the second trimester. You are approaching the delivery date with rapid steps and although you may think that you are done with morning sickness and with all the nasty symptoms that come along with pregnancy, you're not just done yet. As a matter of fact, there is a series of further changes you should expect seeing and you should definitely be prepared for them as well. Read on and find out about the most commonly encountered and about the most important ones.

You May Notice During Second Trimester

- *Still have fatigue*

- *Still have constipation*

- *Still have headaches*

- *Sensitive gums*

- *Ankles and feet start to swell*

- *Decrease in urinary frequency*

- *Increase in appetite*

- *Belly increasing in size, and clothes getting tighter*

- *Fetal movement during the second trimester*

Stretch Marks and Itchy Belly

One of the first things you will notice to change about your body during the second trimester is your belly. With that baby bump will come stretch marks and the feeling of itchiness as well, and this is largely due to the fact that your skin will stretch itself to the maximum to accommodate the new size of your uterus. The sad truth is that there is no way you can prevent the stretch marks to appear. Of course, some women don't get them, but this is apparently related to a genetic

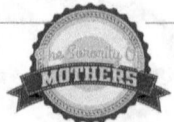

predisposition rather than to anything you can do. Embrace them and accept your body as it is because those little pink, red, violet or white stripes are the signs you have brought into the world a new life, which is one of the most amazing things a human being can do!

Your Cardiovascular System

As a result of the need to fuel your body with extra blood, your doctor may notice an increase in the blood volume in your body. Also, your blood pressure can go down a bit during the second semester and this happens because the blood vessels will basically relax more to allow the new blood volume to flow through properly. It is thus a normal (and good) sign if your blood pressure is slightly decreased. However, if you see any rapid and drastic change, consult with your doctor as soon as possible.

Your Breath

As mentioned in the previous chapter, most of the women experience shortness of breath during the first 3 months of pregnancy. This symptom can be felt during the following 3 months as well. You may feel as if you're not getting enough oxygen and your breathing rate may increase a bit. This is both because your body is trying to get used to its new condition and to provide you with enough oxygen and because the expansion of the uterus may press upon other internal organs (including the diaphragm).

Your Back Pain

As your belly grows larger, you will start bending forward even more. This may alter your body's sense of balance. You may continue (or just start to) feel back pain and the best way to try to counteract this is by trying to have a correct posture (or at least as correct as it can get).

Hand Pain

This is quite rarely encountered, but some women develop hand and wrist pain due to the fact that their bodies retain more fluid, which presses upon the nervous system. This is called the "carpal tunnel syndrome". In very few of the cases women who develop this syndrome may require surgical intervention, but other

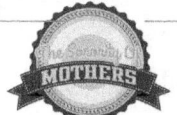

than that you will be able to get through this by using wrist supports and by avoiding any kind of repetitive movements.

Leg Swelling

As your weight goes up, as your posture changes and as your body starts retaining more water, you will most likely experience leg swelling. However, if you ever feel that one of the legs is more swollen than the other one or if one of the legs is more painful than the other one, you should definitely talk about it with your doctor. Some women develop deep vein thrombosis during their pregnancy and this means that the blood clots and that there is quite a large risk for it to break off and to travel to the heart.

Your Gums

This may appear to be an odd one, but did you know than at least half of the women out there experience-bleeding gums during their second trimester? This is quite normal, considering the fact that the hormonal changes will basically send more blood towards your gums and they will become more sensitive. Your gums should stop bleeding once you deliver though.

Congestion, Snoring and Nosebleeds

Again, this may appear to be odd to you, but your nose will most likely congest during this trimester. This is a result of the hormonal changes will make mucus to line the nostrils. As a result of congestion, you may start snoring at night as well and some women experience nosebleeds too. However, if you want to use a decongestant, make sure that you consult with your doctor first and that you bend on the more natural choices out there.

Your Feelings

Many women start to get cold feet as they notice that the delivery date is approaching. It is perfectly normal to feel anxious, nervous or even scared, but same as with the mood swings that sometimes appear during the first trimester, you should always make sure to talk about these feelings with someone. Your mother, a friend who has already had a baby, your spouse or anyone else willing to listen can help you shed off some of these fears at least.

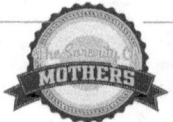

Maternity Clothes

Not all the pregnant women out there are very happy about maternity clothing and if you are among them, then you will want to postpone the moment for as long as possible. The good news is that you can get "away" with wearing loose clothing and pants that don't have anything that may hurt your belly, especially if you are not delivering multiples. Your baby bump will be noticeable, but if you really don't want to wear maternity clothing, you should be able to wear normal clothing during this trimester.

Hemorrhoids

While many people don't understand how exactly pregnancy could lead to the development of hemorrhoids, the truth is that many women out there experience this too. Mainly, this happens due to the fact that the large blood flow and the pressure of the uterus may make the small blood vessels around the anus grow swollen.

Varicose Veins

Due to the large blood flow as well as due to the extra weight your feet will have to carry around, the blood circulation in your lower part of the body may suffer and as a result your veins may become blue or purple. Furthermore, spider veins sometimes develop too, but it should all come back to normal once you deliver your baby.

Baby Moving

The second trimester is the time when you may start to feel your baby slowly moving into your uterus. It is normal if you don't feel it already though, since many of the women start experiencing this only towards their 6th month of pregnancy.

Outside of all these symptoms, there are many other that may appear. Some of them are actually symptoms that were described in the previous chapter. While morning sickness may disappear after the first trimester, heartburn, constipation, headaches and other such symptoms may stick with you into the second trimester as well. All these symptoms are normal.

However, if you feel extreme dizziness, if you bleed or feel severe abdominal pain or if you notice that you are not putting on enough weight or that you are putting

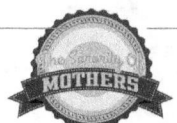

on too much, then you should definitely consult with your doctor. In most of the cases, a ½ pound to 1 pound every week is the normal weight gain pregnant women should experience. If you notice that you have put on less than 10-20 pounds during the entire second trimester or if you notice that your weight gain goes beyond 6 pounds/week, you should also make sure to talk to your doctor about it.

Pre-term labor can appear in the second trimester as well and it is of the highest importance that you know how to tell the signs. Basically, pre-term labor is defined by the dilation of the cervical area and by regular contractions. This entire situation can be very, very dangerous for the baby so if you start feeling these symptoms, call the emergency service right away. Still, do keep in mind that having irregular contractions is quite normal and commonly encountered out there and that they don't pose the risk the pre-term labor contractions do. These ones will be irregular in frequency, strength and duration as well.

In addition to the contractions, you may experience other symptoms that may be an alarm signal for the fact that pre-term labor has installed. These symptoms include: pain (somehow similar to the gas-type ones), low pelvic pressure, vaginal bleeding, excessive vaginal discharge and pain in the lower back area. You don't need to worry and obsess over the possibility of pre-term labor appearing because this kind of stress can damage the baby's health. Yet, be aware of the potential symptoms and contact a doctor if you are worried that you may have started noticing some of them.

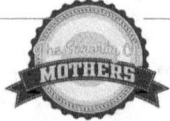

The Third Trimester and What You Should Expect Now

Here you are! Your final 3 months of being a pregnant mommy-to-be!
The first obvious thing everyone will notice is that you will be getting bigger and bigger with every week that is approaching the delivery date. It is normal to feel slightly confused, scared and nervous (and maybe even more than before, since the due date is closer than ever).
Aside from the huge belly, there will be a series of other things that will happen to your body at different levels. While you should not worry about them and while you should not stress yourself out over these things, you should still be familiar with what is very common to happen out there.
Some of the symptoms and things that appeared and happened during the first and second trimester will continue in the third one as well (back pain due to changing your gravitational center and posture is one of them). Other symptoms will be slightly new. Although you are slowly getting closer to the delivery moment, your body will still be making some "last-minute" adjustments, so you should definitely make sure to inform yourself properly over this matter.

What to Expect During Third Trimester

Now that you are at the end of your pregnancy, you should be excited to see your little one and hold them. But you are only is your seventh month of pregnancy, so you have two more months to go. Unless you have the baby early. In the last year or so, the baby being born early has dropped by 3% so you don't really have to worry too much about have a preterm baby.

Now in the third trimester you will start seeing your doctor once a week. While there the doctor checks to see if you dilated any or not. Some women dilate to 1 cm and don't go beyond that for a few weeks or more. While others tend to go from 1 cm to 10cm without really know anything until the doctor checks them out.

- *Healthy Appetite*

- *Some pain in abdomen*

- *Continual Constipation*

- *Gums may continue to be sensitive*

- *May experience leg cramps*

- *Should have increased fetal activity*

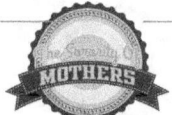

• *Backaches*

• *May have skin changes on the abdomen*

• *Your abdomen may itch*

• *May start to experience hemorrhoids*

• *May experience varicose veins*

Sleep Deprivation

You've got a large body and, most obviously, a large belly as well. This means that sleeping will become a bit of a luxury in most of the cases. For once, it will be uncomfortable to sleep in any position at all. Even more than that, your emotions may be such a rollercoaster by this point in your pregnancy that sleeping may just not be an option.

To top everything, there are specialists who clearly advise pregnant mothers to sleep on their left side only, especially during the third trimester. Apparently, sleeping on your back can damage the oxygen influx of the baby and sleeping on the right side may not be a very good option either. Thus, all you've got left to do is trying to get used to sleep on the left side.

Going to the Doctor

Outside of the cases when you really need a medical professional's advice your consultation frequency will increase as well. Basically, he/she will definitely have to take your blood pressure every two weeks and he/she will have to monitor your body and any kind of changes happening to it.

Contractions

Pre-labor can still get installed, but small kicks coming from the inside of your belly are perfectly normal. While it may be difficult to differentiate between actual labor and the "fake" kind, you should to learn to distinguish them. You will most likely find yourself calling your doctor much more often than before and that is so because you will want absolutely everything to be all right.

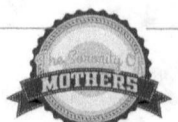

Discharges

Discharges are common in all the trimesters of a pregnancy, but things can get quite confusing when it comes to third one due to the fact that there are many types of discharges women may notice.
The first one is similar to what you have been noticing until the current stage as well. The consistency of the normal vaginal discharges during pregnancy in this trimester can vary a lot, from very thick to watery. This type of discharge can appear as a result of a wide range of reasons. An increase in the cervical mucus substance production can lead to thicker discharges, for example. Also, when women notice watery discharges, they believe that their water may have broken, but in most of the cases this is just the result of your uterus pushing down on your bladder. However, to make sure that everything is all right, if you notice that the discharge has made your underwear feel wet or moist, call your doctor and talk to him/her about this.
Another type of discharge you may notice is the one produced by an infection. It is quite easy to spot if you are experiencing this because the odor of this kind of discharge will most likely be foul. If you have developed a vaginal infection, your doctor may prescribe you antibiotics, as they are considered to be safe to be used during the last stage of pregnancy.
Also, pregnant women in the last trimester can notice a pinkish type of discharge as well. This is a sign that your labor will start within days (and sometimes even sooner) and it is the result of the mucous plug dislodging. If you experience this, then make sure that you are ready to enter your labor.

Pre-Eclempsia

Not many people out there know it, but there are certain conditions that appear only during pregnancy. Pre-Eclempsia is one of them and it is a type of high blood pressure associated especially with the last stage of pregnancy. Basically, it will manifest itself as swollenness, but its onset will be very rapid and the severity may be quite high. So, if you notice that you have become swollen out of the sudden, consult with your doctor immediately.
In most of the cases, the doctor will have to run some blood tests and some urine tests to see if there is a high concentration of protein in your urine or if there are other signs of pre-Eclempsia in your blood. If you are diagnosed with mild pre-Eclempsia, you will most likely be advised to rest in bed and that should be enough. However, if you are diagnosed with severe pre-Eclempsia, your doctor may want to induce your labor because the only cure known to this condition up to the moment is the delivery of the baby.
Again, this is not meant to scare you off, but you should really be prepared for anything that may come along. Pre-Eclempsia is usually more commonly encountered with women who are somehow at the extremes of the normal

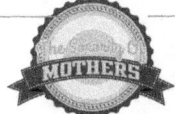

reproductive age (they are either teenagers or women in their late 30s or early 40s). Also, it is more common with first-time mothers as well.

Bleeding

While it is normal to notice spotting during the first trimester of the pregnancy, it may be the sign of a serious issue during the last trimester of pregnancy. Make sure you call the doctor as soon as you notice this happen because it can be a sign of the fact that the placenta grows inside the cervix, of the fact that the placenta has separated from the uterine wall or even of pre-term labor.

Braxton Hicks Contractions

This is a kind of contractions that can appear both in the late second trimester and in the third trimester as well. Basically, they are the irregular type of contractions that has been talked about in the previous chapter. They will not increase in intensity and the duration between them will not decrease such as in the case of the "real" contractions. In one-way or another, this is your body's way of "teaching" you how labor may feel like. In many cases, Braxton Hicks contractions develop into actual labor so it is important that you notice if the timing between two contractions becomes considerably lower.

Breast Discharge

As you approach the delivery date, you may notice how your breasts are considerably larger (up to 2 pounds, actually). Also, you may notice a yellow-like fluid that leaks from your nipples. This liquid will actually be your baby's food for the first days of life, so it is perfectly normal if you notice it (and it is a very clear sign that your body is ready to deliver the baby).

Various Symptoms

There are many cases in which symptoms that have started developing during the first trimester of pregnancy will continue appearing during the second and third one as well. Back ache, shortness of breath, frequent urination, hemorrhoids, heartburn and constipation – all these things are quite related to the size of your belly so you should not expect them to "vanish" away after a specific week or trimester. In fact, it is quite likely that they will get more and more poignant as you approach your delivery date.

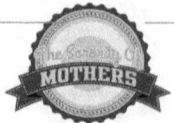

Pregnancy Health Red Flags

Most of the red flags women may encounter during their 9 months of pregnancy have been touched upon throughout the previous chapter, but it is definitely worth to bring them together in one place only, so that you can actually have them in handy.

Vaginal Bleeding

As it has been mentioned before, a lot of women notice blood spots on their underwear during the first trimester. However, if you notice any kind of larger bleeding, it is high time you contacted the emergency service as soon as you see this. Any kind of vaginal bleeding that doesn't resume to some spots during the first trimester can be a sign of a health problem and it is not to be taken lightly.
Bleeding can be a sign of miscarriage, of an extra-uterus pregnancy, of an anomaly in which the way the placenta grows, of pre-term labor or of a placenta that has torn itself apart from the uterus walls – all of which are very serious conditions that can very seriously affect your health and the health of the baby.
In general, problematic vaginal bleeding is associated with a series of other symptoms as well: abdominal pain, cramps, lightheadedness (and even fainting), lower baby movement rate and so on. Listen to your body and go to the doctor as soon as you feel that something is not all right!

Baby Movements

During the second trimester of pregnancy, most of the mommies-to-be will feel their babies moving for the first time. While some of the women experience this earlier into the second trimester, others experience it much later on (almost into the third trimester), so if you are past your 5th month and haven't felt it yet, don't worry – it will come to you as well.
It is extremely, extremely important that you listen to your baby. Whenever you feel that he/she is not moving as usual, contact your doctor immediately because you really want to make sure that everything is all right with you and with the baby as well. Also, if you feel that your baby is moving much more violently than the usual, contact the emergency service too.

Blurry Vision

If you start having blurry vision, if you start seeing "spotty" or if you have any kind

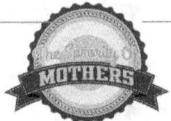

of vision-related symptoms, make sure to contact your medical professional immediately because this could be a sign of pre-gestational diabetes (a kind of diabetes developed during pregnancy and which can go away once the baby is delivered) or a sign of pre-Eclempsia (a condition that has been talked about earlier as well).

Severe Headaches

It is normal that you have headaches, especially during the first and second trimester of pregnancy, when your body is still trying to adjust to the huge changes it is going through and when hormones will have it their way. Yet, if you feel that the headache will not go away in any way, if you feel that you cannot concentrate because of it, if you feel that it is very severe, make sure you are consulted by a doctor because this could be, again, a sign of pre-Eclempsia.

Swelling

Swelling is very normal in pregnancy, but if you notice anything that is just too much make sure you get yourself to the doctor as soon as possible. Especially when swelling is associated with headaches, dizziness and other such symptoms, it is very important that you receive medical attention because it could be a sign of pre-Eclempsia or even of Eclempsia (which can lead to organ damage).

Excessive Itching

Again, itching is quite normal during pregnancy, as your skin is stretching itself to make room for the expansion of the uterus. However, if your itchy feeling becomes excessive, always make sure that you visit a doctor because it could be a sign of a liver condition such as obstetric cholestasis. OC, as it is sometimes referred to, is usually associated with pale stools and with dark urine as well.

Vomiting and Diarrhea

While it is quite common that pregnant women vomit (especially during the first 3 months), if you notice vomiting or diarrhea that have become excessive it is of the utmost importance that you receive medical attention because these symptoms can lead to severe dehydration and when that happens, the baby cannot get sufficient nourishment either.

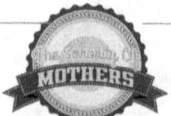

Fever

There is no rule saying that pregnant women cannot catch the flu, but the truth is that fever can be a sign of an infection as well. If you notice fever and none of the other typical flu symptoms (runny nose, coughing, sneezing and other similar symptoms) you should definitely seek medical help. If your fever is higher than 99.5 degrees F, you should seek extensive care. If the fever goes even higher than 102.2 degrees F, you will need emergency care.

Contractions

Generally speaking, most of the women experience contractions when they enter labor (the "real" contractions, not the irregular ones). However, there are certain circumstances when contractions are not normal. For instance, if the pregnant woman is having regular contractions long before the expected delivery date, it is important that she goes to a hospital. When contractions are associated with vaginal bleeding as well, you should make sure to call the emergency service. If you notice that your water has broken down and it has an odd color (yellow, green and so on), make sure you call 911 as soon as you notice this. Also, if you feel that you have to push or if you feel that the contractions are very intense, but you are not expecting yet, you should definitely call the emergency service as well because this could be a sign of pre-term labor.

Pink Fluids before the Due Date

Usually, leaking pink fluids means that you are most likely approaching labor and that you will enter it within days or less. However, if you notice this kind of leak before the term (2, 3 weeks or even much before that), you should make sure to contact medical help because you may enter pre-term labor and you will need medical assistance.

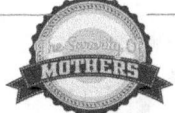

How to Maintain Yourself Healthy

Your health and the health of your baby are very, very tightly connected. You really have to make sure that you take care of your body because Junior will be counting on you to do this and you really have to be very careful with every single move you make from multiple points of view. Here are some tips on maintain you and the little one inside of you healthy and strong so that you can have a normal delivery and a healthy and happy baby.

Your Condition Before Getting Pregnant

It is a very clear fact that mothers who are healthy and fit before they get pregnant have more chances of delivering a healthy baby and, if you have decided that you want to have a baby, then do make sure that you adjust yourself to this wish. That means that you should start embracing healthy habits as soon as possible because they can really change everything for you and for the baby as well.

Eat healthy, exercise and keep yourself health in general. If you smoke, quit it. Don't drink excessive amounts of alcohol (and don't drink any of it during the pregnancy). Don't make excesses of any kind. Keep yourself balanced, healthy and confident and by the time you get pregnant, you will have less to work on when it comes to adjusting to the needs of your baby.

Cat Litter and Toxins

There are some pregnancy-related myths out there, but the one that says that pregnant women shouldn't change cat litter is not a myth at all. Actually, you should stay away from your cat's litter as much as possible because there is the risk of toxoplasmosis, an infestation that is caused by a parasite. While adults who get infested with it will think they are just having a flu, this kind of medical condition can be very dangerous in the case of children and in the case of pregnant women, since it can cause miscarriage.

As for general toxins, keep yourself away from them at all times. They are not normally good for your body, but since you will be carrying another person in you and since this little person is relying on you to keep him/her healthy, you should make sure that you don't stay near toxins (and this may include hair dyes and hair perm solutions as well)

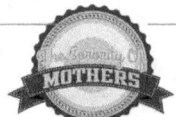

Also, make sure that if you are decorating the nursery room, you will not be the one hanging out near paint and wallpaper because the fumes associated with these will most likely not be healthy for you as a pregnant woman.

Listen to Your Body

If you need to sleep, then go lie yourself down. It is absolutely normal that pregnant women feel very tired, especially during the first 3 months of pregnancy and if you feel like napping in the morning, afternoon and then sleeping all night, then listen to your body. There will come a time (when you will be past your 6th month of pregnancy, for example), when your belly will not allow you to sleep as much and as comfortably as you would want to and when that time comes you will look back and regret not having listened to your instinct.

Water!

Drink at least 8 glasses of water every single day. You need to keep yourself hydrated now more than ever because your body really, really needs it. Dehydration can put you to danger and it can endanger Junior as well. You are allowed to drink other liquids as well, but you may want to keep soda and coffee within normal limits because they contain caffeine and/or they contain too much sugar (both of which can damage your health and, consequently, the health of your baby).

Take Classes

From prenatal Yoga to childbirth classes, there is something for every single stage of pregnancy you will be at. Pregnancy exercises, early pregnancy classes, Yoga, childbirth classes, breastfeeding classes – all these things are very good to attend to because they will really prepare you for what is to come. Even more than that, they are a good way of coming in contact with a lot of people who may help you with information, with advice on where to find a good hospital and other such matters.

Stretch, Tilt and Keep Good Posture

You will be carrying a lot of weight in your belly and your entire body may start bending forward. To make sure that you won't be extremely bothered by back pain later in the pregnancy, make sure to stretch your arms and your back, to tilt your

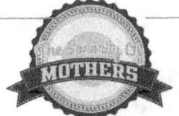

cervical bone and to keep a generally good posture for as much as you can. Small changes such as these ones can really make the difference eventually.

Prepare Yourself Psychologically

Nobody said bringing a little person into the world will be easy and truth be told, the 9 months ahead of you are just the start. In fact, you are about to change your life forever and nothing will ever be the same because you will have to bear the responsibility of a little human who needs you for care, education, health and so on. Make sure to prepare yourself psychologically. At times, you will feel downright terrified of what is to come. Other times you will feel excited. But no matter what happens, you will still love being a new mom and you will want to cherish every single minute.

Talk to Your Baby, Listen to Him, Read about Other Birth Stories

It is very important that you keep yourself positive and that you send the same energy towards your baby bump as well. Believe it or not, while the baby may not fully understand you, he/she will get acquainted with your voice and this is where the unbreakable connection begins.

Also, it does help if you read the stories other mommies out there go through and it helps if you have a more experienced mommy to talk to because many of the fears and anxieties can be alleviated this way.

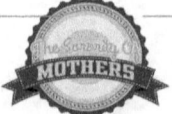

Pregnancy Health Issues

Outside of the symptoms most of the women experience, there is also a series of illnesses and medical conditions that are typically associated with pregnancy. Again, some of them have been mentioned under the different stages at which they may appear, but since you will most likely want to keep them in mind, it is worth bringing them together into an entirely different chapter as well. So, here are some of the diseases and medical conditions frequently associated with pregnancy (and which not many people who never had a baby actually knew of):

Eating Disorders

If you were suffering from any kind of eating disorder when you got pregnant, make sure that this disorder will not affect you and your baby during the pregnancy. Women who suffer from eating disorders have been shown to have a greater risk of bearing babies with birth defects and prematurely, so make sure that you know what you do if you have even a mild version of anorexia or bulimia (take into consideration the fact that your body image will change as well so your disorder may aggravate as you continue with your pregnancy).

Depression

Women who suffer from depression before getting pregnant will most likely suffer from it during the pregnancy as well. Even milder forms of depression can affect the way in which you look after yourself (and thus, after your baby), so do make sure that you talk to someone if you feel that sadness is overwhelming you.

Diabetes

Women who suffer from diabetes at the point at which they get pregnant may not know that most of the doctors advise those in the same situation to get the diabetes under control with at least 3 months prior to trying to get pregnant. This is extremely important because the fetus can be harmed by the high levels of glucose in the blood.

Asthma

This is quite commonly encountered out there, but pregnant women should be especially careful with how they manage their condition. Poorly managed asthma

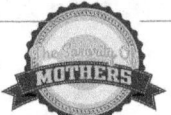

can have serious repercussions over the pregnancy: pre-Eclempsia, insufficient weight gain for the fetus, having to give birth through a C-section and many other complications that can get very, very serious. Even if you have a mild form of asthma you should still make sure to get it under control if you get pregnant!

Obesity and Being Overweight

Being overweight before getting pregnant is not just about your health, but about the health of the future baby as well. It has been shown that women who are overweight or obese show greater risk of bringing into the world premature babies or of suffering serious health conditions during the pregnancy themselves (pre-Eclempsia, for example, which can harm both you and the baby and can get extremely serious).

Anemia

As it was mentioned before, there is a special kind of anemia, which is related only to pregnancy. This is mostly connected to the fact that the body will start producing approximately 50% more plasma, but it will produce only about 20% more red blood cells, which can eventually lead to a lack of balance your body will perceive as anemia. If you feel tired, if your skin looks pale or if you show any other typical anemia symptoms, you should visit a doctor because he/she will be able to prescribe you with prenatal supplements that will help.

High Blood Pressure

High blood pressure has been talked about earlier as well and it is one of the main symptoms of what medical professionals call pre-Eclempsia. Of course, not just any rise in the blood pressure will automatically mean that the expecting mother has developed pre-Eclempsia, but if you notice anything odd about your blood pressure, then you should definitely consult with a doctor and see if there isn't anything else that may be going wrong.

Pre-Eclempsia

This has been mentioned in this book before and it is a very serious condition that should not be taken lightly. Its main symptom is, as mentioned above, high blood pressure, but there will be other symptoms associated with it. The swelling of the hands and of the face, the presence of a high level of protein in the urine, dizziness, blurriness, severe headaches and stomach pain are among the other

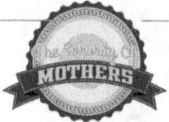

symptoms of pre-Eclempsia. In the case this medical condition is severe, the only cure ever known up to the moment is the actual delivery, so the doctor may suggest a C-section if you are diagnosed with pre-Eclempsia.

Hyperemesis Gravid Arum

Put in plain English, this is a medical condition that develops during pregnancy and which is manifested through severe nausea and vomiting. Morning sickness is normal, but when it becomes severe, you should definitely talk to a medical professional about it and see if there is anything that he/she may recommend or prescribe to help you with alleviating these symptoms.

Placenta Previa

Although not under this name, this condition has been mentioned previously in the book as well. Basically, this condition occurs when the placenta covers the cervix and it can be quite dangerous.

Placental Abruption

This medical condition occurs when the placenta of a pregnant woman separates itself from the walls of the uterus before the due date. This can leave the baby without oxygen so it is important that it gets spotted and that measures are taken so that the baby is fine.

Cytomegalovirus

This is a commonly encountered virus that can affect the newborn baby of a mother who has been infested with the actual virus. In the case of the infested mother, there aren't very strong symptoms (sore throat, mild fever, and swollen glands – symptoms that can be typical of the flu as well). However, in the case of the baby, serious disabilities can appear, such as loss of hearing and vision issues as well.

Group B Strep (GBS)

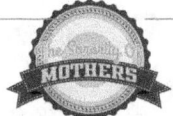

Very commonly encountered in women's vagina and rectum, this bacterium does not affect the adult pregnant woman. However, it can lead to the death of the baby if it is passed in any way during the childbirth.

Listeriosis

This is an infection caused by a bacterium that is found in many readymade and frozen products. It causes fever, diarrhea, muscle sores, nausea and it eventually leads to stiff neck and headaches. In the worst cases, it can lead to premature birth and even to miscarriage.

Parvovirus B19

This virus causes what is known as the fifth disease. This doesn't cause severe symptoms in the case of the pregnant women who get infested with it, but in the worst cases out there it can lead to miscarriage in the first 20 weeks of pregnancy. Typical symptoms include rashness on the face, trunk and limbs, low fever, tiredness, painful joints and so on.

Toxoplasmosis

This is the disease caused by a bacterium that is found in cat litter – which is the main reason pregnant women should not clean their cats' litter. For the woman, it doesn't cause any serious symptoms and it may even pass along as a mild flu. However, if the unborn child is infested with it, severe disabilities can appear: intellectual disabilities, hearing loss, vision loss and so on.

Yeast Infections

These are quite common out there and although they may not cause any kind of serious symptom, they are definitely hard to deal with when pregnant (mainly because no medication that can cure it can be administered to a pregnant woman).

Urinary Tract Infections

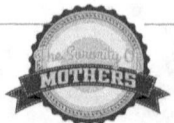

These infections are very common as well, but they can become even more problematic during pregnancy because once spread to the kidneys, it can lead to preterm labor and preterm birth.

The Flu

The common flu (or influenza) can be very dangerous when pregnant because the symptoms caused will be more severe and this can lead to preterm labor and delivery.

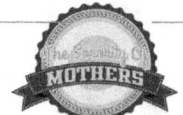

The Final Countdown: The Delivery

If you were expecting things to be as easy as simply going through the 9 months (with their ups and their downs) and then showing up at the hospital, you should think again. Yes, in theory, everything goes according to this plan. But before you even start to approach the final moment when you will be delivering the baby, you should make sure that you are very thoroughly informed on what the delivery will be like and on which are the things you should be taking into consideration about it.

When Do You Actually Go to the Hospital?

Some people out there may answer very simply: when you're in labor. However, for first-time mothers, when and how exactly labor feels like can be quite confusing and they may end up going to the hospital a couple of times before they are actually admitted. So, when do you jump in the car and alert the entire family?

Basically, your contractions will be the ones telling you when it is high time to take your significant other, to pack your bags and to actually get yourself going. If you are having contractions that are regular, that are increasing in intensity and that are very painful, then you need to go to the hospital.

Also, your water will break. Bare in mind that this is not the normal leakage you have been experiencing throughout the pregnancy and that it will actually be like water when it comes to the consistency.

Furthermore, you may start feeling cramps or you may start feeling as if you need to do bowel movements and as if you needed to push. However, it is quite likely that what you are feeling has absolutely nothing to do with your bowels and that you are not yet at the stage when you should really push.

Listening to how your baby moves in your belly can help you determine if you have to go to the hospital as well. Take one hour and count if you get 10 kicks, rolls, turns or whatever kind of movement from your baby. If you don't, see if you can count them in 2 hours. If your baby doesn't make 10 movements in 2 hours, then you should definitely go see a doctor. Also, bear in mind the fact that, as the delivery date approaches, your baby may start to be less and less active, but that will not prevent him/her from making at least 10 movements in 2 hours.

Other than that, your mood may tell you a lot about when the delivery date has come. You may become overly sensitive, you may feel a lot like crying, and you may feel even more scared than before. All these things are very normal,

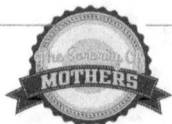

especially with the importance of the moment and with the tons of hormones running through your body at the moment.

If you show some of the symptoms, but you are not in labor yet, the doctor will most likely send you back home. If he/she notices that you are on the verge of entering labor, you may be held in the hospital and you may be suggested to make a bit of physical effort such as walking down the hallways for a bit. If that happens, then you may be able to "induce" labor.

What to Pack for the Hospital?

In the heat of the moment, you may forget a lot of important things at home so it will be better for you if you make your baggage as soon as you see that the due date is approaching. This will save you up a lot of time if you go through your labor very rapidly and it will prevent you from forgetting anything at home. So, which are the things you should be taking with you at the hospital? Here is a list that should give you a broad idea:

- Soap

- Shampoo

- Toothpaste and toothbrush

- Hair brush or comb

- Makeup if you plan on wearing any when you get out of the hospital

- Anything that will make you feel good

- Clothes for you (make sure you get loose fitting clothes such as a dress or even your pregnancy clothes because your weight will still be with you even after the delivery)

- Night gown (make sure you can open it up easily if you will be nursing)

- Slippers

- Robe

- A bra and underwear (make sure that the bra is either one made especially for nursing or one that you have been wearing during your last trimester of pregnancy)

- A gown for the baby

- Blankets for the baby to wrap him/her up

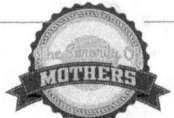

- Bad weather clothes for the baby

- Baby undershirt

- Baby booties

- Car seat

- A video camera to preserve these adorable memories

How a Normal Delivery Will Be Like

If you are associating the word "normal" with "hassle-free", then reconsider your position. A normal delivery will be scary both for you and your spouse and it will be confusing and odd if this is the first baby you are having. Yet, by the end of it, you will be able to hold your little precious in your arms – a feeling you can compare to nothing, absolutely nothing in the world! Here are some of the few things you should know about normal deliveries:

The Labor

Not many of you may be familiar with the fact that there are 3 stages of labor. The first one is also split into 2 different phases: the latent one (when you are very much likely to be sent back home from the hospital) and the active one (where they will take you in the hospital and diagnose your labor). The latent phase can last for anything between a few hours to 14 hours, so be prepared to face whatever comes your way. As for the second phase, you will most likely get through it at a faster pace than with the first one.

The second stage of labor is that of the cervix dilation. When the cervix dilates to a maximum of 10 centimeters, you will be told to push – and this is when the actual birth begins.

The last stage of labor occurs after the actual birth. This is when your placenta will have to come out and it can last up to 30 minutes, normally. At the end of all these 3 stages, you will have given birth already.

Also, you should definitely know the fact that there are cases when the labor may slow down up to the point where it stops completely. If that happens, there could be 3 main causes: an unknown one (dysfunctional labor pattern), the fact that your pelvis is not large enough to allow the baby to pass through or the fact that you may have an infection in the uterus. Doctors will check for the consistency, strength and occurrence of your contractions, they will check the size of your pelvis and they will also check with the position and orientation of the baby

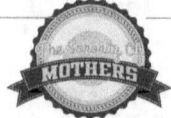

(he/she could, for example, have his/her head turned to an improper position, which prevents him/her from passing through the pelvis).

Labor can be induced, that is true, but doctors will not call for this kind of measures unless you are past due date or if you meet other requirements. Administering medication meant to simulate the labor is one of the most encountered ways of inducing it, but it can come with a risk: failure. If the doctors have failed to induce labor through medication, you will have to undergo a C-section – which is one of the main reasons most of the professionals in this field are quite reluctant to doing it.

Other than that, sex is supposedly a natural method of inducing labor. However, if you can't do this, then you may want to talk to your doctor about it. Other natural solutions include a cervix examination made by the doctor where he will basically loosen what makes the water bag stick to the uterus' walls. If you are properly dilated, the doctor may even forcefully break the water as well, this way inducing the actual labor.

The Hospital

You may be surprised, but even if your labor is very obvious and even if you are diagnosed straight away, things will not be as easy as simply showing up there. Actually, you will be required to sign a lot of forms because even if you are giving birth, paperwork is, well, paperwork. Since you will be *slightly* busy with bringing a baby into the world, your spouse can take of everything BUT he will not be allowed to sign in your place!

Also, you may be surprised at the fact that doctors will not talk "human" language. You may hear something like 4 centimeters, 50% and then some "non-sense" you may not fully understand. What they are measuring is your cervix: the number of centimeters shows how dilated it is, the percentage shows how much it has effaced and the other number will most likely be at what distance the baby's head is from the ischial spines (the bones of your cervix, basically).

Also, even when the medical staff will speak plain English, you may find it difficult to concentrate on what they are saying. Make sure that your significant other or the person who is with you will listen carefully and that he/she will be able to relay everything to you once the delivery process is done.

What Happens Next: Medication and Other Things

Once you are accepted in the hospital, you will be taken to your room. Be prepared for the fact that the nurse may administer certain medications and that

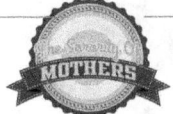

usually means that an IV will be "installed" in your arm. Pain medication, dilation medication (when necessary) and other types of medication may be administered. Also, in certain cases, the woman in labor may need a blood transfusion. Furthermore, the anesthesiologist who will check if your IV is in good functioning will see you, just in case you may need an emergency C-section.

Also, many women wonder whether they will be shaved before they enter the delivery room or not. Indeed, this used to be practiced everywhere out there, but now this is not done any longer because it is believed that it may lead to small injuries that could grow into infections. If you will be having a C-section, your doctor may require shaving, but this is a matter of every medical professional's preference and not a prerequisite anymore.

Pain Relief Options for Child Birth

There are several options for pain relief. There is local anesthesia, regional anesthesia, and general anesthesia. Local means that they numb your vagina with a numbing medication. Regional is things like the epidural, which is placed in your spine in your lower back. Then there is general, which puts you to sleep during.

Delivery Options

Most of the women give birth in hospitals, naturally. Yet, there are at least 3 other options out there and before you even approach the due date, you should take them all into consideration because one of them may be more suitable for you than the other ones. Here are the 4 types of delivery you can choose and what you should know about them:

Vaginal Birth at the Hospital

This delivery option has been talked about previously in this chapter. This is probably the safest and the most natural way to give birth. It may not be the most pain-free one, but this is the main way women have given birth for millennia now and this is the safer way to go.

As soon as you enter labor, you will be admitted to the hospital. You may be given medication (especially to help with pain), but other than that no anesthesia will be administered.

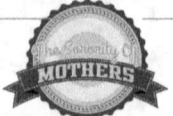

C-Section at the Hospital

Many women would rather go for the C-section because they know that this will happen under anesthesia. Yes, C-section can appear to be a lot "friendlier" than other types of delivery (as it will be less painful and it will prevent you from suffering urine leaks until the vagina recovers to its normal size), but the truth is that it comes with various risks.

For starters, you should know that no matter how "simple" things may appear, a C-section *is* a surgery – and every single type of surgery out there poses certain risks to the person who is on the table.

You could develop an infection (around the cut area, in the womb, urinary tract infections and so on). You could develop a blood clot as well. You could suffer an adhesion (which basically means that one or more of your organs could stick to the walls of your tummy). You could suffer adverse reactions from the anesthetic. You could injure your reproductive system. You could be prevented from giving birth vaginally in the future. You may suffer from things that may affect your future fertility. Even more, studies show that babies delivered through C-section can suffer breathing issues (both if they are delivered before the term and if they are delivered before the labor has actually started).

As you can see, a C-section is in no way something to joke or play around with and you should consider thoroughly if you want to go under the knife from the very beginning. Of course, if there are certain things that may prevent you from delivering normally, the doctors will most likely suggest a C-section themselves, but actually choosing for this should be thought of thoroughly.

Vaginal Birth at Home

Giving birth at home can sound like a wonderful option, especially for those of you who would much rather be in a friendly environment, surrounded by people they love and appreciate – not by complete strangers. Of course, in addition to the friendliness of the place where you give birth, there are other important things to consider as well. For instance, giving birth at home can help you avoid pain killers and medication, it can be helpful for those who know that they have a history of fast labor, it can be a good option for those who have certain religious or cultural beliefs, it can also be a good choice for those people who may want to save up some money, it can offer you with more freedom of movement, of eating what you want during the labor and so on.

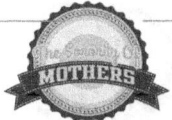

However, if you think that these advantages would appeal to you, and then you should also make sure that this is done properly. You need to make sure that you will have an experienced midwife with you and sometimes even a medical professional will be required. Also, you will have to create a birth plan that will include what you will have to do before, during and after the birth (such as receiving postpartum help, for example).

In case of complications, you should also be prepared to go to the hospital because there are certain things that cannot be done at home (for instance, if you really need to be C-sectioned, it will not be safe to do it at home, but in a completely germ-free environment such as the hospital). Also, you have to make sure that you ask your caretaker as many questions as possible and that you listen to him/her if he/she suggests that a hospital may be better for you.

Furthermore, there are certain situations when giving birth at home is not at all the best solution. If you have a chronic disorder, chronic diabetes, if you have had a C-section in the past, if you show pre-eclampsia symptoms, if you have multiples, if your baby is not well positioned in your uterus, if you are more 3 weeks before the due date or 1 week past the due date - these are the main cases when you should not choose to give birth at home.

Also, there are cases when you should be transferred to the hospital. For instance, if your labor is not progressing at all, if your placenta peels off from the walls of the uterus, if you have vaginal bleeding and if you have any symptoms that are considered to be pregnancy red flags, then you should make sure that you are ready to be transferred to the hospital

Generally speaking, there are no risks associated with giving birth at home (as long as you keep yourself carefully monitored by professionals). Yet, there seems to be a higher occurrence of infantile death and complications in the case of those who give birth at home as compared to those who choose a planned hospital delivery, for example.

Vaginal Birth after C-section (VBAC)

You can have a VBAC if what caused you to have a c-section the first time isn't a problem this time. A VBAC is called Trial Labor After C-section (TOLAC). About 60-80% of women go on the have successful VBAC's.

There are factors that make you a candidate for a VBAC. Those factors are that your incision was made horizontal and not vertical. Pelvis seems to be large enough for the baby to pass through.

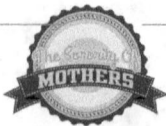

There also things that can keep you from having a VBAC. Those factors are being an older mom (over 35). Having a high BMI, having a high birth weight (8.8 lbs.), having your pregnancy goes over 40 weeks, and also having a short period before getting pregnant again (less than 18 months.)

Vaginal Birth In Water

This has become quite a popular option these days, but if you don't really know if it is really the best one, then you should make sure that you inform yourself properly and that you consider both the advantages and the disadvantages connected to it.

You can choose to labor and/or give birth in the water and one of the main pros of doing this is related to the fact that water will make you feel easier and that it will alleviate pain without the need of medication. Furthermore, there is a lot more privacy and there is a lot more freedom of movement, both of which are considered to be very important advantages by many of the ladies out there. You will also most likely be pushing easier, since the water will make you sense this as an easier task. As for the baby, it is believed that the passing from the mother's womb to the water pool is easier on him/her than passing from the cozy motherly "home" to the hospital room's air.

Of course, there are disadvantages to laboring and giving birth in the water as well. For instance, some women who labor in water have been disappointed by the fact that their labor did not actually start or if it progressed too slowly. Also, there is the risk of an infection (which actually exists in the case of the hospital delivery as well). Pain may be relieved, but it will not be completely inexistent, as many women believe water laboring is.

As for giving birth in the water, one of the main risks is associated with babies who start breathing under water. Most of the babies have something called "dive reflex", which means that they will automatically hold their breaths. However, if you deliver the baby's head before the rest of the body, if there is some sort of problem with the oxygen in your placenta or if the baby is startled during the birth, he/she may breathe in. Your midwife should be able to prevent all these cases, as much as it is in his/her power.

Also, there may be issues with the umbilical cord. Once the baby is born, the midwife will bring him/her to surface as soon as possible and this rapid movement sometimes causes the umbilical cord to snap. However, this is not a very hard to deal with situation if your midwife is actually well trained.

As you can see, there are many ways in which you can give birth and you should definitely choose the one that suits you. Remember that while some women may

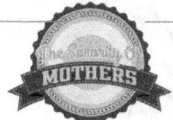

feel great with the idea of giving birth under water, for example, you may not be as comfortable as them. If an idea simply doesn't appeal you in any way and if you are ready to take in the risks of trying something else, then follow your instinct because it may just be the best advisor. Put everything in balance and make sure you don't rush into a particular decision.

There are some women who do their plans for delivering their baby and they want a water birth. The women who do water birth have to go without pain medications because if they are in the water with pain medications, it could stall the labor. For the early stages of labor the mother-to-be has to stay out of the water because there is a change the water will also cause the labor to stall as well.

When the woman is allowed into the water, the water covers everything up to her shoulders. There are several ways to ease the pain. Those things are meditation, guided imagery, and hypnosis.

Normally water births are done with a midwife. There are several types of midwives. There are CNMs, CMs, CPMs, and DEMs. CNM stands for Certified Nurse-Midwife, CM stands for Certified midwife, CPM stands for certified professional midwife, and DEM stands for Direct-Entry midwife.

CNMs have at least a bachelor's degree. CMs are college educated and certified by ACNM. ACNM stands for American College of Nurse-Midwives. CPMs are certified professional midwives who are certified by NARM. NARM stands for North American registry of midwives. DEM stands for direct-entry midwives. Those have trained through apprentice.

What to Buy For Baby: The Essentials

Now keep in mind that you may or may not feel you need everything that says you need for the baby. So here is a list to look through:

- Packs of diapers
- 1 pack of disposable wipes
- 6 drool bibs
- 3-5 wash clothes
- Thermometers
- Brush and comb sets

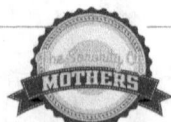

- Crib or pack n play
- 5-8 bottles
- A bottle brush
- Stroller
- Swing
- Changing table
- Dresser

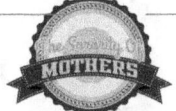

Taking the Newborn Home: Things You Have to Know

Once everything is done and if both you and your baby are in good health, you will be allowed to finally come back home with your little cupcake. After 9 months of seeing your body grow, change (sometimes in odd and unpredictable ways) and after several months of feeling your junior playing football in your belly, you will be finally HOME.

Leaving the Hospital

Before you leave the hospital, make sure to dress your baby accordingly. Many overly protective mothers feel the need to wrap up their babies until they can't actually see them anymore. However, overdressing your infant will not be a good choice. That crochet hat you made for your little baby boy or baby girl may look awfully cute, but if it's summer and hot outside, he/she will most likely feel terribly uncomfortable with it. A cotton shirt and some pants should do. If it's winter outside and if the weather is bad dress your baby in appropriate clothes for the season and then wrap him/her in a blanket.

As it was mentioned previously as well, one of the most important things you will really have to have with you will be a baby seat. No state out there will ever allow you to transport your bundle of joy from hospital without a safety seat, so make sure to buy a good one. Infant-only seats are really better and more suitable for newborns than convertible seats so you may want to buy one of those first. Also, you should ALWAYS place the seat in the back of the car and NEVER in the front. Also, DON'T hold your baby in your arms! It may feel that he/she is safer this way, but the absolute truth is that he/she will be much, much better off in the child seat because that is where a baby is the safest. Not only do you risk a huge fine for not respecting the legislation, you risk something even more importantly: the health and safety of your baby – and that is not something to fool around with no matter what happens!

What to Have Home

Also, you may want to make sure that everything you will need for the following days will wait for you at home. This will not only help you have everything in handy when you need it, but it will also help you feel more comfortable with your new situation as the mother of a newborn.

Make sure you will have a cradle and some extra blankets and sheets, make sure that your baby will have enough onesies and gowns to be dressed in and make sure that the nursery room will be clean and well oxygenated. Also, make sure you prepare everything you will need for breast feeding if you choose to do that

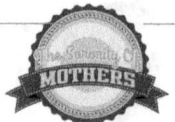

(ointments for the nipples, breast pads and so on) or that you will have everything you need for formula-based feeding (the formula, several types of bottles to see which one will be more appreciated by your pumpkin, and so on).

If your baby has undergone circumcision, make sure that you have everything that is needed to take care of him. Also, remember to put on the must-have list the products you will be using for your baby's umbilical care as well.

A notebook can be very helpful because jotting down bowel movements, sleeping hours and all these details can help you adjust your schedule from now on as well. Also, you may want to have a baby album and a camera to keep those precious memories intact (and to embarrass your baby when he/she turns 21, of course).

Last, but definitely not least, remind yourself that you really, really need to stock up on diapers. Lots of them. Your baby may be small and you may underestimate how many diapers he/she will need during this first stage, but the truth is that he/she will actually use them... a lot.

Other than that, bring in all those things that make you feel comfy: a pillow (maybe even a doughnut pillow), magazines (you won't have any time for reading, but anyway), some snacks (you *will* be hungry and you *will* want something nice to crunch on), some comfortable clothing and so on.

What Other Things to Expect

If you thought that those odd feelings would simply go away once your cupcake is delivered into the world, then you were wrong. You will still feel scared and overwhelmed with emotion and you may still want to run away and scream as loudly as possible.

Also, do bear in mind the fact that post-partum depression is something as real as it gets and that you will want to make sure that you know how to deal with it in case it starts developing in your case as well. Many moms feel sad and confused after giving birth, but if your feelings of depression are quite severe, then you most likely suffer from post-partum depression.

It is important to acknowledge this and to seek help in those you love and even in professionals that may help you with counseling. It is important that you know that this is not a flaw and that there is nothing wrong about you having these feelings. After all, you have been through a lot *lately* and post-partum depression installs the same way as a birth complication – it will not be your fault.

Postpartum psychosis is an even worse psychological condition that is characterized by paranoia, hallucinations and confusion. In some of the cases, mothers want to hurt themselves and/or their babies and in case a woman is

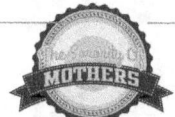

experiencing such symptoms immediate help should be sought for. Postpartum psychosis is not very common out there, but you should definitely know about it because it is a real thing and because anyone can be affected by it.

Another thing you may not have thought of is related to the fact that your baby will need regular medical checks. Make sure that you arrange this with your chosen pediatrician before the delivery time approaches. If you haven't yet made any arrangement, talk to the hospital doctors because they will be able to guide you in this matter. They will be able to tell you when the first routine check should take place and where you should seek for help in this. These checks are absolutely essential because they will monitor the development of your baby and they will help you and the doctor spot anything that may not go as well as it should be in due time, so that it can be fixed.

Also, another thing you may want to consider is the way in which your pets will welcome the newborn. If you have a dog, you should make sure that he somehow gets accustomed to the baby even before you introduce the two of them to each other. Some of the people choose to take one of the baby's blankets and give them to the dog so that he can get used to the scent of the newborn. This way, the baby will not feel like a stranger for your pet and he will not perceive your pumpkin as any kind of threat. Ideally, this should be done before you leave the hospital so ask your partner or significant other to bring home the blanket as soon as he/she can get his/her hands on it (the sooner the pet gets acquainted with the little one's special smell, the better it will be when you come home).

Another thing many parents do not consider when it comes to their newborn baby is related to the fact that, well, everyone will want to see the little bundle of joy and they will all want to visit. Since you have been through birth giving and since you probably didn't have the best 9 months of your life with all the changes you went through, you will most likely not be able to entertain everyone. Even more, it is important that you limit the number of visitors your baby gets every day because, believe it or not, your pumpkin can get tired of too many strangers waving and giggling at him/her.

Even the most sociable babies will need to sleep and they will not be able to get their much-needed rest if everyone keeps "bugging" them. As for you, you most likely need your rest as well. It is OK to tell people that you may not be able to accept visitors for a while and to tell them that you will receive them as soon as you get accommodated to your new situation. After all, this is your health and your baby's health and you really need to take care of both.

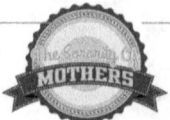

Calling the Doctor

Many new mothers (and fathers as well!) feel overly protective towards their newest member of the family and they feel that they should be calling the doctor whenever something out of the ordinary happens. Don't get this the wrong way: you really need to call the doctor if you notice anything suspicious – but make sure you don't do it because the baby had one incidental itch or because he had one quarter of a teaspoon of milk less than the day before.

On the other hand though, call the doctor as soon as soon as you notice any of the following issues:

- High rectal temperature (anything above 100.4 is high)

- Dehydration (no wet diapers for more than 6-8 hours, crying without tears, feeling a depression in your baby's soft spot in the head and so on)

- If your baby is not very easy to rouse

- Bloody stools, bloody vomit

- Breathing difficulties (this is an absolute 911 situation so don't waste any time with asking yourself whether or not you should be calling the emergency service!)

- Diarrhea stools (more than 8 in 8 hours)

- A bulging soft spot

There will be other things as well that should make you call the doctor. Following your instinct is a good idea under these circumstances and if you really feel that something is wrong with your baby, do press the call button because you really want to make sure. Your doctor will not mind it – after all, that is his/her job and he/she probably knows how scary it can be to be a new parent and to be so confused and not to know what to do when your baby cries (and even more so if they ever had babies of their own).

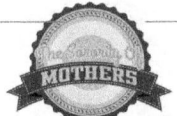

How to Make It through The First Months

Pregnancy and delivery are just the beginning of a long and beautiful journey that will never actually end. Once you are a parent, you will always bear the responsibility for your child's wellbeing and the truth is that this is the most wonderful job anyone out there can get.

The first few months of being a parent will be tough on both of you (on all three of you actually). Sometimes, your baby may cry and you may not be able to tell why and how you can help him/her. Other times, you will want so bad to see those magic firsts (such as the first laughter) that they will come only when you expect it the least.

There are some things you may want to keep in mind when it comes to how to take care of your newborn for the first few months of life. Of course, an entire library could be written on this, but this chapter has aimed at bringing together the most important tips on newborn parenting.

Don't Expect to Sleep Much

You may not actually expect this, but it will be difficult to get a full night of sleep during the first months of being a mother, the same way as it was difficult to sleep when you were going through your last months of pregnancy.

The key to getting through with this is to stop obsessing over the fact that you are tired. Yes, you are and everybody will believe you if you tell them – and even more so everyone else who has had a child already. Instead, focus on caring for your little bundle of joy and make sure that you truly offer him/her your best because the bond that will be created now is hard to break.

To make sure that you keep yourself sane and as healthy as possible, make a plan with your significant other to take shifts. This way, both of you can get at least *some* sleep and both of you can care for the baby as well.

Also, try to see how your baby will sleep and when are the times at which he/she sleeps the best and the most – those will be your sleep hours as well. Believe it or not, that sweet giggling creature in the cradle will set the alarm clock and an entire day's schedule for the rest of the house as well.

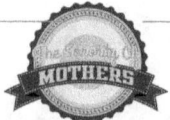

Soothe Your Baby

As mentioned, it will sometimes be difficult to actually tell what your baby needs. One of the best ways to go is to try and fail and then try again – soon enough, you will be able to "translate" "baby language" and you will learn how to take better care of your little strawberry cupcake.

One of the things to do is to always try to mimic the womb, both when it comes to the position in which you hold your baby and when it comes to the movements you make. Shushing, swinging and all these things can help the baby feel better. Believe this: the passing into this whole new world is tiresome for the little one as well and he/she will need some time to get used to this new home and this new life.

Warm baths can be OK, but you will want to do this only after the baby's umbilical cord has fallen off. Also, warming things up (such as the towels you use to wipe your baby's diaper area) can help too.

Furthermore, try soothing music as well. Babies like music and it will help both of you relax and soothe your psychological state, your bodies and your souls. Also, if you find anything else that works; try to remember it and to use it again in the future as well.

Getting Help

Sometimes, you will feel like breaking down. The responsibility of taking care of a baby that cannot actually tell you what is wrong with him/her can feel like the entire burden of the world has fallen on your shoulders – and you are not to be blamed for this.

However, when you need help, do ask for it. Try to involve your significant other in taking care of the baby, but if he/she doesn't feel comfortable with it, then do not press too much. Friends and other relatives of yours can actually help a lot if you allow them to.

However, try not to listen to any kind of piece of advice that may sound too confusing or too overwhelming. Instead of listening to old midwives' tales, inform yourself properly and learn things from people with hands-on experience. If any kind of advice feels fishy, make sure that you follow your gut instinct.

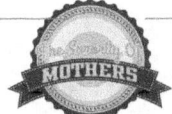

Taking Walks With Your Baby

At a certain point during the first months, your doctor will tell you that it is safe to take your pumpkin out in the world. When you do this, always make sure to take everything you may need with you.

Do not forget about diaper changes, about taking a spare blouse or T-shirt to change in if your baby has some *fun* with your current clothes, and about all the other things you know you use often. Also, try to take a more experienced mommy with you and try to only go to places where children are more than welcomed. This way, you will prevent yourself from finding yourself in odd situations and you will not feel alone either.

Being Overwhelmed

Now, lets say it has been a week or two. You are exhausted from getting up with the baby every few hours at night. Then you can ask family members, who are not busy, if they could come over so that you could get some sleep. Most family members would jump at the chance to see the baby, especially grandparents. If anyone offers to help you, don't turn him or her down because eventually you are going to want any help that is offered.

Family members know what its like to have a newborn in the house and how stressed out mommy and daddy could be. When it comes to newborns, they cannot have full-blown baths yet. Until the circumcision (If you have a boy) heals up and the belly button cord falls off, they will have to take sponge baths.

Postpartum Depression

It may be one of the most difficult things to deal with and the most unexpected as well. Postnatal depression is one of those medical conditions that few understand. Not only does this tend to catch many women off guard, but also even doctors aren't always prepared to help. There is so much wonderful anticipation of a baby arriving and when that moment comes, many women expect to feel nothing but joy. As with any other aspect of pregnancy or parenthood however, there are often some rather unexpected elements that come up and that must be dealt with.

It's important to note that this is a very serious health condition and should be dealt with appropriately. Though postnatal depression used to be quite misunderstood and therefore misdiagnosed, it is taken very seriously within the medical community. You need to discuss this condition with a doctor even during your pregnancy so that you understand the symptoms.

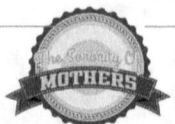

This isn't something that happens to "other women", this is a condition for which you have no control over and for which there is a great deal of help available. So though you may feel as if this condition is something to feel bad about, this is a very common condition that you can receive a great deal of help for.

The problem is that it hits many women without warning. Just as a woman feels that she is finally able to embrace this new chapter in her life and love and adore her new little bundle, the hormones and emotions take over. This is very frustrating and disheartening and may even be brushed off because most women want to believe that this can't possibly happen to them.
The reality is that many women feel this on varying levels and therefore the time to move forward and determine if there is something going on is right away. You can get help, you can get back to normal, and you can enjoy your new little baby but you have to first recognize what exactly is going on. That's often the hardest part—admitting that something is wrong in the first place!

We are going to take you through a journey and discuss what to be on the lookout for. We are going to help you to understand the steps, the symptoms, and how to cope with it all. This isn't something to be taken lightly and though it affects women on varying levels, postnatal depression is something that should be prepared for in advance just in case it happens to you.

Let's start by recognizing that this condition doesn't mean that there's anything wrong with you. This has nothing to do with your amount of love or adoration for your newborn. This condition has everything to do with your hormones, your body adjusting to birth and life after birth with a newborn, and it can even come on due to lack of sleep or nutrients or other basic fundamental needs. So knowing this in advance can really help you to feel prepared and to cope with the situation if you are in fact somebody that suffers from postnatal depression.

Know too that not everybody feels the effects of this in the same way. You may know of a friend or family member who had a very mild case where they felt a bit sad or blue and that was the end of it. You may even know of somebody on the other end of the spectrum who struggled and spent months feeling bouts of crying and even anger. Just know that no two cases are the same and so you should be prepared for the unexpected.

Postnatal depression doesn't affect everybody, but it is something to be aware of. You may go through your pregnancy with ease and then find that the months after baby's arrival are the most difficult. You may make it through the first few months with nothing at all. If nothing else, there must be greater awareness for postpartum depression and so this book will help to highlight what to know and how to get the help that you may find that you need.

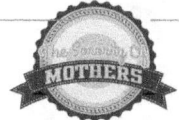

Understanding Postnatal Depression

One of the biggest problems with postnatal depression is complete understanding the condition. This is a condition that for many years was misdiagnosed or ignored because the medical community and society in general really didn't have the knowledge required to help. Many women suffered through the symptoms and the depression and it made for a very rough transition into motherhood. The sadness was confused with an adjustment period and therefore doctors and even friends and family just stood by while women suffered from the symptoms.

Fortunately there is so much more information out there about postnatal depression. This has become such a common condition that many doctors discuss the symptoms and likelihood of postnatal depression with their patients even during pregnancy. This isn't meant to scare women but rather to prepare them and to help them to be on the lookout for the telltale signs. This is all a positive thing as women are finally getting the help that they have needed for so long.

It's often hard for people to understand why postnatal depression occurs. The birth of a child is supposed to be such a positive and wonderful experience. Some women wait their whole lives for this or go through difficulties in conceiving and so it doesn't seem natural that they are filled with sadness after the birth occurs. Many don't want to believe it and therefore the misconceptions and ill information tend to come to the forefront because it's not the way that it's "supposed to be".

No woman wants to go through postnatal depression but it is more common than you might realize. Just as no pregnancy is the same, no postnatal period is the same either. Even with your own pregnancies you may suffer from absolutely no symptoms at all with one pregnancy and then find yourself lost in the depths of depression with your next. So know that you are not alone and that many women have gone through the same sentiments and symptoms that you suffer from. To some that offers comfort alone and therefore an understanding of what this health condition is all about.

Getting to the Heart of the Issue

We'll discuss the ins and outs of postnatal depression but first there must be an understanding of the condition itself. Knowing what it's all about can help you to be aware of it and therefore recognize if you are going through it. Some women find that being prepared for the potential onset for postnatal depression can be of

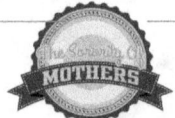

great help in this already transitional time period of their life.

Some important things to know about postnatal depression include:

- *It often starts with a feeling of sadness:* Though you are feeling hormonal and exhausted you may blow off your feelings of sadness. This is very common because most women don't want to believe that they feel sad during a seemingly happy time. Though a bit of sadness may be nothing, this is often the first sign and something to keep tuned into. If the sadness continues or worsens then it may be necessary to get some help or to talk to your doctor.

- *It can be confused with a lack of sleep or difficulty adjusting:* Sure you are going through a major transition in your life and that's all normal. The problem arises however when you are exhausted, have a difficult time in adjusting, can't seem to bond with the baby, or are feeling sad more often than not. If you are feeling hopeless or find that the adjustment is more than you can handle or that you even anticipated then that's when it is something more and likely that you are suffering from some level of postnatal depression.

- *It is usually present within the first few months after the baby arrives, but can be present for a year afterwards*: What many people don't realize is that the symptoms of postpartum depression can come on and linger for over a year after baby arrives. This means that you may be suffering months after the arrival and have the symptoms and not even realize it. So this is not just a condition limited to the first couple of months, but rather is something that is present and possible to contend with for a year or even beyond in extreme cases.

- *Many women don't want to admit what they are feeling or don't ask for the help that they need:* There is no shame whatsoever in admitting that you feel the symptoms of this. As a matter of fact it's admirable to get help and it is very common. So the reality is that you must recognize that if sadness or even hopelessness is present or if you are having a hard time bonding with baby or can't stop crying, you need help. No matter how subtle or extreme the presence of this condition

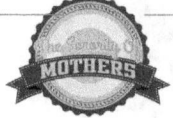

may be, know that it's imperative to get help and to never be afraid or ashamed to admit you are suffering from the condition. Postpartum depression is a very real medical condition and must be dealt with and diagnosed properly to get help and allow the woman to get back to normal.

About the Sorority of Mothers

www.asororityofmothers.com

Is a gathering place for mother to share tips and experiences with ONE MISSION, to make being a MOM easier for all future mothers and experienced alike. We are constantly working on new books and topics that can help our members and readers. There is not instruction manual for being a mom!

Motherhood

Defined as the state or experience of having and raising a child. Raising a child today is much different than raising a child 10, 20, or even 30 year ago. Technology, society, and social media are just a few different elements that either aide or harm motherhood.

Knowledge is power. Maternal instinct can be boosted with knowledge. Knowledge is the core purpose of the Sorority. With our growing membership, we are creating a mastermind of mothers. All with different backgrounds and experiences. The whole is greater than the sum of parts.

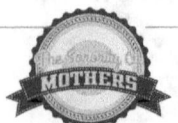

Become a member
You can join easily by clicking the button below.

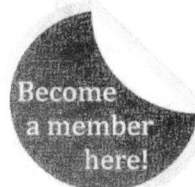

Enter your email address, we will be in contact and will send you a free book of your choice as a gift for your membership.

Contact Us
asororityofmothers@outlook.com

Like Us on Facebook, click the like icon
https://www.facebook.com/asororityofmothers

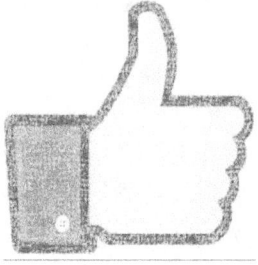

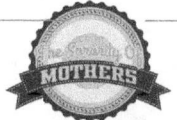

Preview: The Ultimate Week by Week Pregnancy Handbook

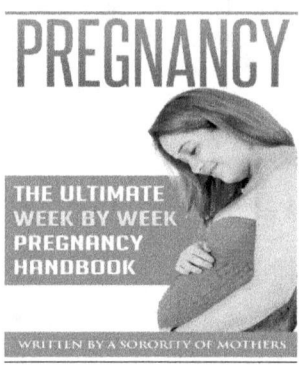

Finding Out You Are Pregnant

You may have had a vision for how that special moment would go for years, and now it's here. The moment of truth, the moment you figure out if you are in fact pregnant. For many women this is a moment that they have planned for and are anxiously awaiting. There are fair shares of women who are shocked or surprised by their pregnancies, and so sometimes preparation isn't always a factor.

No matter what your situation, that moment when you find out that you are pregnant can be quite magical. Though you may or may not have expected it, there is something about seeing that positive pregnancy test that is almost defining. It can set the tone for a wonderful pregnancy through the ups and downs and really help to solidify this next exciting chapter of your life. But first you have

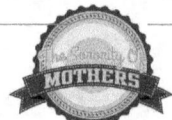

to get there, and embrace the step of finding out that you are in fact pregnant.

Sometimes that positive pregnancy test is the only surefire indication that you are in fact pregnant. While some women can tell early on, others need that positive test to show that this is what is going on with them. Everyone is different and therefore the beginning stage and very early weeks can be a completely individual experience. Though you may not be like your friends in the way that you find out that you are pregnant, there are a few helpful things to keep in mind.

As you begin your pregnancy and ensure that you are in fact with child, consider a few factors into the big picture, such as:

Look for the telltale signs if they are present: For some women they can tell that something is different within their bodies. It may be as obvious as a missed period or it may be something a little subtler. They may feel exhausted, may have headaches or breast pain or other symptoms. Recognize that the first couple of weeks can be early for symptoms overall, but it is certainly possible. If something seems different or if you are late for your period, then be aware of this. These early signs may present themselves if you are looking for them, though not all women will get the indication like others.

Take the pregnancy test at the right time: Though you may be tempted to take the pregnancy test right after you believe that conception occurred, this can actually backfire. If you take the test too early it can result in a negative because the hormone levels aren't high enough to be indicated just yet. You want to be sure to be patient for as long as you can and take the test at the exact right time. There are some pregnancy tests that can now detect pregnancy as early as a few days before your next cycle is due and that may work. If you want to be absolutely certain though wait until you have officially missed your period and then take the test. This is where tracking your cycle's can really come in handy!

Know that sometimes the beginning can be a little slow: While some women may exhibit those symptoms of pregnancy that we mentioned, others may not have any indication whatsoever besides a positive pregnancy test. So if you are feeling nothing out of the norm or having no symptoms there is no need to worry. As you will see in the next chapter, the vast majority of symptoms don't usually present themselves until much later on when the hormones are in full surge and the baby begins to really develop. So if you feel nothing, don't worry or think that there is anything wrong, as no two pregnancies are alike!

Give yourself time to process: Even when you are prepared and anxiously

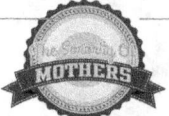

awaiting a pregnancy it can be a lot to take on mentally. Do give yourself some time to process this big news and to live with it. You are about to become a mother and this is so exciting and yet so scary at the same time. Give yourself time and room to feel what you need to feel and know that it will continuously change and evolve as you move forward with your pregnancy.

Figure out how to share the excitement: When it's time to share the exciting news this can make for a really great reveal. If possible try to put a bit of creativity into telling your husband that he's going to be a dad. Tell family and friends in your own unique way and on your own terms. There is no right or wrong way or time to tell people that you are pregnant and this is a very individual thing. Do it in a way that works best for you and by all means have fun sharing the excitement. That's one of the best parts of this early stage.

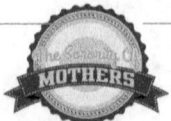

The First Couple of Weeks and Coasting: Weeks 1-7

So you have confirmed that you are pregnant—congratulations! Now comes the exciting time, right? Well to be honest those first few weeks are a time that many pregnant women find to be a bit uneventful. Though you may be frustrated that things aren't moving fast enough for you now, just wait as things will progress quite nicely as you move forward. Some would tell you to enjoy this quiet and somewhat comfortable time.

In your first pregnancy you have no idea what to expect or what to look for, and so you examine each and every element of your life and may even worry. Know that though things may not change much now, that's not really a bad thing. Your body is getting used to its new state and it may take a few weeks to sort of catch on. You may find that many symptoms don't fully take shape until about the eighth week of pregnancy, and that is extremely common.

The first seven weeks or so can be a time for what some may refer to as "coasting". This is a time where the baby is just starting to take shape, the hormone levels are starting to begin their climb, and your body is just starting to get used to its new pregnancy. This means that for many women there are no telltale signs and therefore they may worry that the pregnancy is not real. Though this is a common concern, there is usually nothing at all to be worried about.

Once your body starts to grasp what is going on and the baby starts to grow, there is plenty of time for the signs to show up. You may be wishing back upon this quite time, as some of the symptoms such as nausea, headaches, and the general uncomfortable part of pregnancy becomes a reality.

So if you are worried about what these first few weeks are going to be like, consider a few key tips that can help you to adjust and to mentally prepare for what lies ahead. Consider this a quiet and even relaxing time to get yourself ready for the excitement and roller coaster that lies ahead in the next several months of your life.

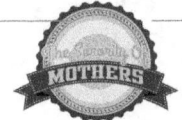

What Do These First Few Weeks Hold In Store?

Consider a few highlights of the first seven weeks or so. This can help to ease your mind, get you prepared, and help you to learn to enjoy this quiet and often uneventful first stage of pregnancy.

Schedule your first doctor's appointment: Once you find out that you are in fact pregnant through a positive test you want to call your OBGYN's office. They may have a set timeframe as to when they want to see you, and this may be anywhere from 6-8 week of pregnancy. They will ask you the date of your last period to detect how far along you are and so you want to have that in mind. The first appointment can be very reassuring for many women and so it's great to get this set and to go in with any questions that you may have in advance.

Be patient and know that it may take time for signs to show: Again some women have symptoms the minute that they find out they are pregnant or even before, but this isn't the norm. For many women it takes a bit of time for the body to catch up so be ready for that waiting period. Don't worry if you feel no different or see no changes in the body. Everyone is different and every pregnancy is different and you just might be the lucky one that gets away with a symptom free pregnancy—or it just might take a few weeks to kick in completely.

Be aware of anything to look out for: Though there is usually nothing to worry about at all, do be on the lookout for anything unusual. If you have cramping, bleeding, or anything unusual or alarming then call your doctor right away. Though many women worry about these things happening, most have no reason, as this will never be an issue. If something worries you then by all means have it checked out just to be sure that nothing is amiss—doctors expect pregnant women to call with concerns.

Try to enjoy the "calm before the storm": Embrace this time in your pregnancy because it will pass very quickly. Soon enough you will have plenty of symptoms, your body will be changing, and your baby will be taking over. Get into good habits during this time period and take good care of yourself with eating the right foods and getting plenty of rest. Know that there is much excitement ahead and if you get a bit of quiet now that's a good thing!

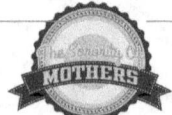

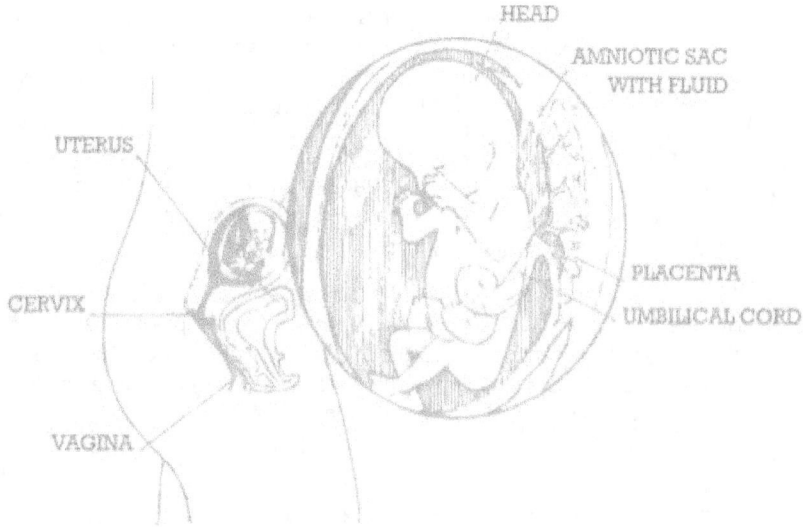

UTERUS

HEAD

AMNIOTIC SAC
WITH FLUID

CERVIX

PLACENTA

UMBILICAL CORD

VAGINA

The First Trimester

It is the first trimester of your pregnancy from the minute that you find out that you are pregnant. The truth is however that you may not actually feel pregnant until about the eighth week. The reason for this is that you surely aren't showing just yet and you aren't going to really feel much in the first few weeks. There's something about a symptom kicking in or actually seeing the baby on an ultrasound that tends to solidify it for most moms.

You can expect with many doctor's offices to be seen for your first appointment somewhere around the eighth week. This is a magical time as you have everything confirmed, and though you knew you were pregnant it just feels far more real at this point in time. This marks a very big milestone, particularly when you have a doctor's office that will in fact do an ultrasound at that first appointment as additional confirmation.

Every doctor will vary, some will see you sooner and some may wait to do a first ultrasound. It's really up to the discretion of their office, and so you should ask.

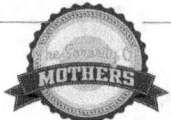

The first appointment however is a great time either way to ask pivotal questions and to see what exactly is going on with the pregnancy and with you. There are a lot of changes starting to happen, which the least of is missing your first period and the magic and madness continues from there on out.

For some women they don't really feel pregnant until they are showing. For others though that first trimester when things really start to kick in and feel real makes for a magical and wondrous time. You can try to get prepared for this, but in the end it's all about experiencing it for yourself.

First time mothers often feel that the first trimester is a time when it seems to go from zero to sixty in no time at all. One day you don't feel pregnant at all and then the next you have symptoms or signs of pregnancy galore! So be prepared for some magic and some changes to start happening in this pivotal part of the first trimester marking the beginning of pregnancy overall.

Weeks 8-12: When the Symptoms Really Kick In

Though there is a great deal of magic happening around the eight week and on it can also be a time of frustration. While you may feel great about the fact that you can tell that you are pregnant, at this point in time it usually comes in the form of symptoms. We all know that there is a great possibility that symptoms may be a part of pregnancy, but it's almost unexpected in some way. You tend to be overwhelmed when these symptoms come about as they are all too often out of the blue and hit you with a bang.

There is nothing to fear because as quickly as these symptoms come about they tend to go away just as fast. You may feel completely weighed down with exhaustion or even nausea one minute and then it's gone the next. Most women who experience substantial symptoms tend to feel them within the first trimester, and they are often gone at the beginning of the second trimester. So though it may feel like an eternity, you can hopefully expect the symptoms to go away in just a few weeks.

So what kind of symptoms can you expect around this timeframe? The good news is that the backache, frequent urination, and constant uncomfortable feeling aren't usually part of the first trimester symptoms. The types of symptoms you can however expect to experience include but are not limited to the following:

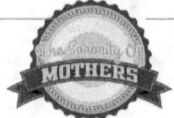

"Morning Sickness": This is probably the most misnamed symptom of pregnancy. Though some women may experience morning sickness in its truest form, others will not feel their nausea until they reach the evening. It's all about the hormones and the baby's development and the way that it hits you. It may be that you feel nauseas and want to throw up but never do. You may be somebody who throws up every day without any relief. It may just feel as though you are on a boat going up and down. There is no rhyme or reason and when that nausea hits just do your best to try and relax and stay calm, and know that it too shall pass.

Headaches: The constant changes in the level of your hormones makes for some pretty nasty headaches at times. That's the most common reason for headaches in the early stages and therefore they can feel debilitating. You can take some over the counter pain relief if you need to. If the headaches are due to fluctuations in hormones then know that they will pass once you reach the second trimester.

Exhaustion: This is the symptom that nearly every pregnant woman can identify with because it seems to happen to everyone. Consider the fact that you have raging hormones, your body is changing, and you are building another human within you and it's really no wonder that you feel completely drained. Many pregnant women describe this exhaustion as a complete worn down, tired, and drained feeling like they have never experienced before. You will get some energy back in the second trimester when you are usually at your best throughout pregnancy.

Food Aversion: Some women will find that this is the first and most distinguishable symptom of pregnancy. When foods that they would eat regularly sound repulsive such as chicken for example, this is often a telltale sign that something is unusual. There is usually no explaining it except for the fact that the body just doesn't want these foods or even beverages such as coffee, and therefore you will likely keep away from them for the duration of your pregnancy.

Breast Tenderness: You may find that you never have any breast tenderness or that it starts almost the minute that you get that positive pregnancy test. Consider the fact that the breasts are going into preparation mode for breastfeeding and it all makes sense. Some women will say that they can't even handle going over a bump in the road in a car without excruciating pain, while others will feel absolutely nothing. This is a common symptom and it may come and go throughout your pregnancy.

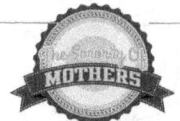

This first trimester is amazing and full of so many wonderful things. As you may suffer through some symptoms know that they will pass soon enough and they just solidify that you are pregnant. Everybody is different though so the type, severity, and frequency of symptoms are sure to vary and that's just fine—all perfectly normal!

As far as baby is concerned by 9 weeks all your baby's body parts will be present but not yet fully formed.   He or she will be about the size of a grape – about 2cm long and weighing about 2g.   He or she will more than double in size over the next 3 weeks.

By 10 weeks your baby will be about 3cm long and will weigh about 4g. All its vital organs – liver, kidneys, intestines, brain and lungs – are fully formed and functional.

By 11 weeks he will have fully formed fingers and toes with tiny fingernails.   His or her genitals will be starting to form properly.

By 12 weeks he will weigh around 14 g and will be about 5.5cm long.   His skeleton is now complete and the bones are beginning to harden.   He will be moving very frequently although you will not be able to feel this yet.

Both the 12 and 20 week scans are becoming more important in helping doctors to identify any possible risks during the pregnancy.

The 12 week scan may look at factors such as the length of your cervix, the blood flow through to the baby and a thorough scan may indicate any risks of an abnormal baby, chromosomal abnormalities, a pre-term baby, a small baby and pre-eclampsia.

You will be weighed, and your family history will be noted in detail – which again will help doctors to predict any predisposition to risks.

You can expect to be given some blood tests to check for numerous conditions such as anemia, Urinary tract infection (UTI) diabetes, HIV and sickle cell that may affect the course of your pregnancy.

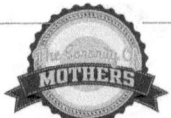

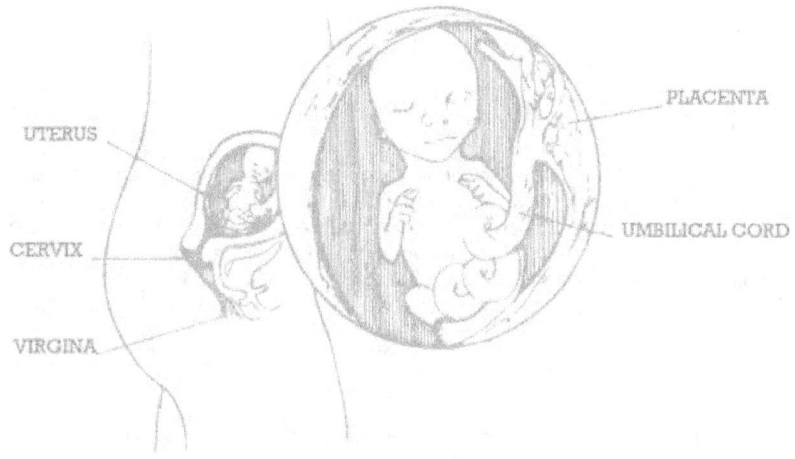

UTERUS

CERVIX

VIRGINA

PLACENTA

UMBILICAL CORD

Buy the book with a click

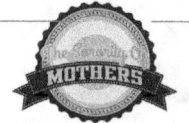

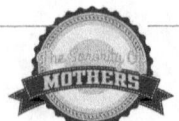

Disclaimer

Legal Notice: - The author and publisher of this book and the accompanying materials have used their best efforts in preparing the material. The author and publisher make no representation or warranties with respect to the accuracy, applicability, fitness or completeness of the contents of this book. The information contained in this book is strictly for educational purposes. Therefore, if you wish to apply ideas contained in this book, you are taking full responsibility for your actions.

The author and publisher disclaim any warranties (express or implied), merchantability, or fitness for any particular purpose. The author and publisher shall in no event be held liable to any party for any direct, indirect, punitive, special, incidental or other consequential damages arising directly or indirectly from any use of this material, which is provided "as is", and without warranties.
As always, the advice of a competent legal, tax, accounting or other professional should be sought. The author and publisher do not warrant the performance, effectiveness or applicability of any sites listed or linked to in this book. All links are for information purposes only and are not warranted for content, accuracy or any other implied or explicit purpose.

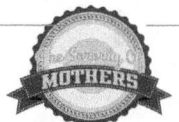